Register Now for Online Access to Your Book!

SPRINGER PUBLISHING COMPANY
C⊙NNECT™

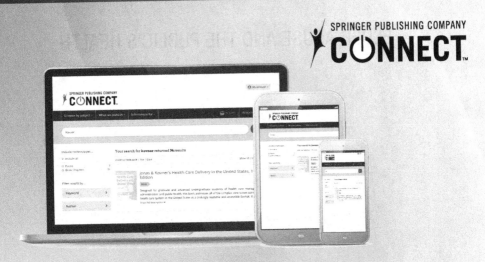

Your print purchase of *Elder Abuse and the Public's Health,* **includes online access to the contents of your book**—increasing accessibility, portability, and searchability!

Access today at:
http://connect.springerpub.com/content/book/978-0-8261-7135-1
or scan the QR code at the right with your smartphone and enter the access code below.

Scan here for quick access.

W8X1XE07

BT

SPRINGER PUBLISHING COMPANY
View all our products at springerpub.com

ELDER ABUSE AND THE PUBLIC'S HEALTH

Pamela B. Teaster, PhD, is the Director of the Center for Gerontology and a Professor in the Department of Human Development at Virginia Tech. She established the Kentucky Justice Center for Elders and Vulnerable Adults and the Kentucky Guardianship Association and was its first president. She is the Secretary General of the International Network for the Prevention of Elder Abuse and is on the Board of Trustees of the Center for Guardianship Certification. She serves on the editorial board of the *Journal of Elder Abuse and Neglect*. Dr. Teaster is a Fellow of the Gerontological Society of America and the Association for Gerontology in Higher Education, and a recipient of the Rosalie Wolf Award for research on elder abuse, the Outstanding Affiliate Member Award (Kentucky Guardianship Association), and the Distinguished Educator Award (Kentucky Association for Gerontology). She serves on the board of the National Committee for the Prevention of Elder Abuse and is a former president. She has received funding from the Retirement Research Foundation, Administration on Aging, National Institute on Aging, Kentucky Cabinet for Families and Children, National Institute of Justice, Centers for Disease Control and Prevention, National Institute of Occupational Safety and Health, Health Resources and Services Administration, and Office of Victims of Crime. Her areas of scholarship include the abuse of elders and vulnerable adults, public and private guardianship, end-of-life issues, ethical treatment of older adults, public policy and public affairs, and quality of life. She has published more than 100 scholarly articles and book chapters and is editor/author of four books.

Jeffrey E. Hall, PhD, MSPH, serves as Deputy Associate Director for Science in the Centers for Disease Control and Prevention's (CDC's) Office of Minority Health and Health Equity (OMHHE). He assists with the provision of leadership and consultation across a broad range of science, research, evaluation, and practice issues to promote the elimination of health disparities and the achievement of health equity. He also conducts research to develop or enhance local, state, and national systems or capacities for measuring and monitoring progress toward health equity.

Dr. Hall was previously a lead behavioral scientist in the Surveillance Branch of the Division of Violence Prevention of CDC's National Center for Injury Prevention and Control. His professional interests include applications of developmental epidemiology and social psychology within violence prevention, structural and environmental methods for reducing violence-related health disparities, and community-based models for violence surveillance, research, and prevention. His work has focused on topics across the life span, including infant homicide, youth and young adult violence, and elder abuse. Dr. Hall is a medical sociologist by training, but also holds degrees in epidemiology, general sociology, and psychology—all from the University of Alabama at Birmingham.

ELDER ABUSE AND THE PUBLIC'S HEALTH

Pamela B. Teaster, PhD
Jeffrey E. Hall, PhD, MSPH

Editors

SPRINGER **PUBLISHING COMPANY**

Springer Publishing Company, LLC
11 West 42nd Street
New York, NY 10036
www.springerpub.com

Acquisitions Editor: Sheri W. Sussman
Compositor: Graphic World

ISBN: 978-0-8261-7132-0
ebook ISBN: 978-0-8261-7135-1

The author and the publisher of this Work have made every effort to use sources believed to be reliable to provide information that is accurate and compatible with the standards generally accepted at the time of publication. The author and publisher shall not be liable for any special, consequential, or exemplary damages resulting, in whole or in part, from the readers' use of, or reliance on, the information contained in this book. The publisher has no responsibility for the persistence or accuracy of URLs for external or third-party Internet websites referred to in this publication and does not guarantee that any content on such websites is, or will remain, accurate or appropriate.

Library of Congress Cataloging-in-Publication Data

Names: Teaster, Pamela B. (Pamela Booth), editor. | Hall, Jeffrey E., editor.
Title: Elder abuse and the public's health / Pamela B. Teaster, PhD, Jeffrey
    E. Hall, PhD, MSPH, editors.
Description: New York : Springer Publishing Company, [2018] | Series: Elder
    abuse and the public's health | Includes bibliographical references and
    index.
Identifiers: LCCN 2018005049 (print) | LCCN 2018011355 (ebook) | ISBN
    9780826171351 | ISBN 9780826171320 (pbk. : alk. paper)
Subjects: LCSH: Older people—Abuse of. | Abused elderly—Services for.
Classification: LCC HV6626.3 (ebook) | LCC HV6626.3 .E428 2018 (print) | DDC
    362.6/82—dc23
LC record available at https://lccn.loc.gov/2018005049

Contact us to receive discount rates on bulk purchases.
We can also customize our books to meet your needs.
For more information please contact: sales@springerpub.com

Printed in the United States of America.

CONTENTS

CONTRIBUTORS

Georgia J. Anetzberger, PhD, ACSW
Consultant in Private Practice
Adjunct Assistant Professor of Medicine
Case Western Reserve University
Cleveland, Ohio

Derrell W. Cox II, PhD
Research Scientist
Center for Applied Social Research
University of Oklahoma
Norman, Oklahoma

Jeffrey E. Hall, PhD, MSPH
Deputy Director for Science
Centers for Disease Control and Prevention
Office of Minority Health and Health Equity
Atlanta, Georgia

James W. Holsinger, Jr., MD, PhD
Wethington Endowed Chair in the Health Sciences
Professor of Preventive Medicine
College of Public Health, University of Kentucky
Lexington, Kentucky

Shalon M. Irving, PhD, MPH, MS, CHES†
Epidemiologist
National Institute of Injury Prevention and Control
Division of Violence Prevention, Surveillance Branch, Morbidity
and Behavioral Surveillance Team
Centers for Disease Control and Prevention
Atlanta, Georgia

Emmanuel D. Jadhav, DrPH, MHA, MSc
Assistant Professor
Ferris State University, College of Health Professions
Big Rapids, Michigan

Lori L. Jervis, PhD, FGSA
Professor
Department of Anthropology and Center for Applied Social Research
University of Oklahoma
Norman, Oklahoma

Elizabeth Podnieks, PhD
Professor and Graduate Program Director
Ryerson University
Toronto, Ontario, Canada

Holly Ramsey-Klawsnik, PhD, LMFT, LCSW
Sociologist/Researcher, Licensed Certified Social Worker, and Licensed
Marriage and Family Therapist
Klawsnik & Klawsnik Associates
Canton, Massachusetts

Pamela B. Teaster, PhD
Director, Center for Gerontology
Professor, Department of Human Development and Family Science
Virginia Tech College of Liberal Arts and Human Sciences
Blacksburg, Virginia

---

† Deceased

Cynthia Thomas, PhD
Senior Program Officer at the Committee for National Statistics
National Academy of Sciences, Engineering and Medicine
Washington, DC

Fatemeh Zarghami, MD, PhD, MPH
Graduate Research Assistant
Center for Gerontology
Virginia Tech College of Liberal Arts and Human Sciences
Blacksburg, Virginia

PREFACE

Although our collegial friendship began more than 10 years ago at a scientific meeting whose name is now lost to us, it would be years before we did more than sit together at meetings. Realizing that elder abuse was both an under-recognized and an underappreciated public health problem, Pamela worked with our kind and patient editor, Sheri W. Sussman, who listened to, and tolerated, too many "dog ate my homework" excuses, including the adoption of a little girl after more than 6 years of waiting. Finally, realizing that "going it alone," even for editorship, was not proving fruitful or providing the depth that the book required (or the fun of producing a book), Pamela approached Dr. Jeffrey Hall about coeditorship. We discussed the idea, and our working arrangement was born—and thus the quality of the book was improved exponentially. Sheri was also pleased with this turn of events and met us both at a meeting of the American Public Health Association to hone the book even more.

Both Jeffrey and I recognized that the time had come to make THE ARGUMENT that elder abuse is a *public health* issue and *the public's* health issue. Although discipline-specific books have been published about aging, healthcare, and human and social services, we decided that the time had come for a comprehensive text that squarely made the proposition, explained it practically and theoretically, and proposed directions for the future. Thus, our goals for this book are fourfold: (a) to establish elder abuse as a public health problem, stressing that primary, secondary, and tertiary preventions of the problem are well within the scope of work performed by public health professionals; (b) to address major public policy/public health initiatives because they relate to elder mistreatment and abuse; (c) to frame elder abuse as a global and human rights issue; and (d) to provide a text that supports the development of core competencies for public health work to prevent elder abuse and mistreatment. The nine chapters of this book frame elder abuse as a public health problem, situate elder abuse and mistreatment within the core functions of public health, and explain elder abuse and the role of public health law and health services administration. From that foundation, we explore elder abuse in the context of topical issues and groups addressed by public health (e.g., intimate partner violence, Native American tribes) and suggest alliances with nontraditional partners. From there, we highlight successful campaigns and model programs that have intersections with public health as well as how elder abuse and public health can and should work on the global stage. We conclude with our synthesis of the central argument of the book as made by its authors and our visioning of future directions for the field.

This book is a labor of love that makes the argument that public health brings unique and important competencies to address the problem of elder mistreatment. The authors of the individual chapters represent an array of diverse backgrounds and expertise. Among the disciplinary perspectives represented are social work, public health, nursing, medicine, gerontology, law, and public policy. The broad assemblage of disciplines is important in adequately addressing an interdisciplinary perspective. One chapter also includes international perspectives.

We do not present this text as inclusive of all aspects of public health as applied to elder abuse and mistreatment. Instead, our book is a polemic about the contribution of public health to elder abuse—one, we hope, that will be an important contribution to the existing literature. Although there are a few texts on the intersection of elder abuse and public health, they do not go into the depth of this book, and rightfully so, because public health is formally addressing the problem in many ways. Yet still, we posit not as fervently as possible and not as deeply as necessary, particularly as concerns the public health workforce at the grassroots level. Our desire is for the text to serve as a useful and reliable resource for those studying and teaching and for those involved in healthcare and public health and human and social services programs. Similarly, practitioners, policy and decision makers, advocates, community leaders, families, and older adults themselves may benefit from this volume.

Pamela B. Teaster
Jeffrey E. Hall

FRAMING ELDER ABUSE AS A PUBLIC HEALTH PROBLEM

Jeffrey E. Hall and Pamela B. Teaster

PURPOSE STATEMENT

The purpose of this chapter is threefold in nature. Its first objective is to fully develop the frame for thinking about, describing, and discussing elder abuse (EA) as a public health problem. This objective is pursued by describing the burden of EA, its societal costs, and the whole of its consequences for public health. The chapter's second objective is to frame EA as the public's health problem. This particular reframing effort is explicitly intended to move the public's perceptions beyond seeing EA as one of many problems confronting society abstractly. Our goal is to achieve acceptance of EA as a problem that we, as members of the public body, must all confront and as a threat that should not be ignored, dismissed, or left for someone else to handle. The chapter's final objective is to introduce a third frame within the field of public health itself, characterizing EA as public health's problem. This aspect of the chapter is wholly inward facing. In this section of the chapter, we argue that EA is a constellation of problematic behaviors that the field of public health must own, contend with,

---

Disclaimer: The findings and conclusions in this chapter are those of the authors and do not necessarily represent the official position of the Centers for Disease Control and Prevention.

and help eliminate for practical, ethical, and moral reasons. We believe the problem of EA fits squarely within the purview of public health as "what we as a society do collectively to assure the conditions in which people can be healthy" (Institute of Medicine, 1988).

ELDER ABUSE IS A PUBLIC HEALTH PROBLEM

EA refers to "any intentional act or failure to act by a caregiver or another person in a relationship involving an expectation of trust that causes or creates a risk of harm to an older adult" (Hall, Karch, & Crosby, 2016). The acts and behaviors globally captured by the term EA have been categorized into several subtypes. These most commonly include physical abuse, sexual abuse, psychological abuse, financial abuse, and neglect. In this conception, the term *older adult* refers to any person whose chronological age is 60 years or older. EA has been framed or portrayed as a public health problem for several decades. The adoption of this framing reflects not only the innate characteristics of this problem, but also the motivations of those advocating its prevention and elimination.

The Innate Characteristics of EA

In terms of characteristics, EA has been justifiably considered a public health problem because it has the potential to affect the health of a large proportion of the U.S. population. The most recent national level, population based study to establish the prevalence of EA indicated that approximately 11.4% of older adults may experience EA (Acierno et al., 2010). When this prevalence estimate is applied to the most recent estimates of the U.S. resident population by age to more concretely illustrate the possible magnitude of this problem, the number of older adults who may have suffered EA in 2014 is approximately 7,388, 265 (U.S. Census Bureau, 2015).[1] This estimate is approximately 14 times greater than the upper enumeration estimate for the size of the U.S. public health workforce (516,193) most recently reported by the University of Michigan Center of Excellence in Public Health Workforce

---

[1] For illustration purposes, this calculation assumes that the prevalence of EA has remained constant during the time since these prevalence data were collected.

Studies (2013).[2] Stated plainly, for every one person in the U.S. public health workforce, there may be approximately 14 persons who may have experienced EA. Within this context, EA is not simply a health problem experienced by just a few persons, but rather a widespread problem that affects the lives of many older adults residing in a variety of places and settings around the nation. In addition, the problem is not confined to the older adults who experience it; the older adults are at the center of a problem that touches the lives of affected others—families and friends, organizations, and society as a whole are all touched by the abuse in tangible and intangible ways.

EA causes segments of the older adult population to suffer harm, injury, loss, and, in the most unfortunate cases, death. The impacts of exposure to EA are extensive and diverse, given that its perpetrators frequently inflict more than one type of EA upon their victims (Ramsey-Klawsnik & Heisler, 2014). Moreover, the impacts of different types of abuse accumulate over time additively and multiplicatively, increasing the likelihood that and extent to which various domains of health will be compromised (e.g., cognition, physical functioning, socialization). The severity of the effects of EA is too often conceived in a disconnected fashion where its respective physiological, psychosocial, and economic consequences are described abstractly and as if they occur separately (Ramsey-Klawsnik & Heisler, 2014). EA's status as a public health problem, however, is further accentuated when it is borne in mind that older adults commonly experience polyvictimization, which occurs *"when a person aged 60 or older is harmed through multiple co-occurring or sequential types of elder abuse by one or more perpetrators, or when an older adult experiences one type of abuse perpetrated by multiple others with whom the older adult has a personal, professional, or care recipient relationship in which there is a societal expectation of trust."* (Ramsey-Klawsnik & Heisler, 2014)

Older adults subjected to EA and those who are concerned about their well-being may have to simultaneously contend with any or all of the following types of abuse, among others:

1. Cuts, bruises, and fractures after having been degraded, humiliated, and isolated from their friends by adult children

2. Coercive, controlling behaviors by guardians who have stolen heirlooms that have been passed down through generations of

---

[2] For illustration purposes, this calculation assumes that the size of the public health workforce in the United States in 2014 is roughly the same as its size in 2012.

family members and who threaten them with institutionalization if they dare tell others about what they are experiencing

3. Overmedication and sedation at the hands of caregivers who misuse prescription drugs to lower or remove capacities to resist or reject unwanted sexual contact and who may dismiss complaints as attributable to delirium or cognitive impairment

4. Frailty associated with deprivation caused by a grandchild's constant failure to provide adequate meals and access to fresh drinking water, indifference to insulin injection abscesses, and restriction of movement to a single small, cluttered room

Such experiences represent just a small sample of the universe of incidents and enduring population-wide patterns of EA that may simultaneously or sequentially produce impairments of cognitive, emotional, physical, physiological, interpersonal, and social functioning and affect the ability of older adults to satisfy their needs for safety, security, social connection, and respect. Insults, violations, and harms occur across these dimensions of health, so the actual and possible undesirable consequences of EA are far greater than most typically acknowledge or contemplate. A phenomenon with so many diverse forms, facets, and health implications cannot be effectively addressed by small groups of individuals on a case-by-case basis, regardless of whether they use intervention efforts or prevention efforts. Therefore, EA has been rightfully promoted for treatment as a priority for societal action that demands comprehensive initiatives, strategies, and resources (addressed systemically in Aravanis, 2002; Bonnie & Wallace, 2003; Connolly, Brandl, & Breckman, 2014; Dong & Simon, 2011; Institute of Medicine & National Research Council, 2014).

The economic toll of EA has also been an element of the frame construing it as a public health problem. This element has been quantified mainly in two ways: healthcare/direct medical care costs and losses associated with financial exploitation. The most current sources place the annual estimated costs of EA at approximately $8.2 billion, with more than $5.3 billion of this cost attributed to direct medical costs and the remaining $2.9 billion representing assets lost because of financial exploitation (MetLife Mature Market Institute, 2011). Other nonmedical costs of EA can include, but are not necessarily limited to, (a) expenses for legal, counseling, mental/behavioral, therapeutic, and rehabilitative services; (b) productivity losses; and (c) costs of funding court proceedings, incarceration, victim compensation processes, and the provision of adult protective services and crisis/emergency response services.

Elders who have been abused have a 300% higher risk of death when compared to those who have not been mistreated (Dong et al., 2009). Although EA-related costs are likely under-reported, elder financial abuse costs older Americans $2.9 billion per year. Yet, financial exploitation is self-reported at rates higher than emotional, physical, and sexual abuse or neglect (Acierno et al., 2010). Estimating the items in the nonmedical category of costs is extremely challenging and has not been successfully accomplished to date. Nevertheless, the high direct costs of EA referenced here are acknowledged as underestimating the true societal costs of this problem. Both medical and nonmedical costs are considered diverted costs, as funds and resources used to address EA could be used to address other needs or desires among individuals or invested in community or societal development efforts. It is important to recognize that these costs are likely to escalate sharply as the proportion of older adults in the U.S. population continues to grow. According to the U.S. Census Bureau, in 2050, the population aged 65 years and older is projected to be 83.7 million, almost double the estimated population of 43.1 million in 2012 (Ortman & Velkoff, 2014).

These characteristics of EA have been presented in reference to three criteria commonly used to define occurrences as public health problems. In summary, EA is a common, prevalent phenomenon; detrimentally affects both individual older adults and large segments of the older adult population of the United States in a variety of ways and at all levels of the social ecology; and exacts a considerable financial and economic toll. The framing of EA as a public health problem using a narrative that includes the aforementioned elements has become common practice throughout the field developed to address EA. This frame now coexists and is frequently used in combination with other frames, such as those depicting EA as a social problem, a crime, or an elder justice issue. Its development and use have helped to alter general misconceptions that EA occurs infrequently, primarily takes place in nursing homes and other long-term care facilities, is a problem relegated to families, and can be addressed only through deterrence-oriented strategies.

Advocacy Motivations

Most stakeholders—groups that can affect or that will be affected by EA or EA-related initiatives—use the frame of EA as a public health problem with three primary goals in mind: (a) encourage others to view the problem as serious and noteworthy, (b) attract attention to and achieve legitimation of the problem, and (c) obtain adequate resources to support actions to address it. With respect to the first goal, many in the U.S. general population are still largely unaware that EA is a problem that our society is currently facing. Although EA was first identified in developed countries, where most of the existing research has been conducted, anecdotal evidence and other reports from some developing countries have shown that it is a universal phenomenon (World Health Organization, n.d.). There is an abiding need to "awaken" groups who are not aware of EA's health impacts and enlist their aid in confronting this problem. Many stakeholders frame EA as a public health problem to inspire thought about the acute need for action, why movement is necessary, and the dire consequences of inaction for our loved ones, communities, and nation, both now and for future generations.

Turning to the second goal, the framing of EA as a public health problem has also been carefully crafted to attract the attention and arouse the interest of both the general public and specific actors. Details regarding the need to obtain acceptance of this issue by the public are provided in the next section of this chapter. Specific actors from whom attention is overtly sought can be collectively labeled "decision makers." These decision makers are public or private persons, entities, or bodies with the authority or capital to (a) place EA on legislative, administrative, fiscal, practice, or scientific agendas to ensure that it achieves and remains an action item; (b) identify relevant goals for efforts to address EA; (c) recommend and/or select specific actions to be taken; and (d) decide which organizations or units will implement selected initiatives, policies, programs, or practices. Decision makers also include agencies, boards, or committees that determine whether authorized actions will receive resources, the levels of resources to be made available, and, in some cases, how the appropriate resources can be deployed. Some stakeholders have framed EA as a public health problem to secure its acceptance and treatment as a priority by a wide array of decision makers. This has involved legitimation processes that not only seek acknowledgment of the need to address EA, but also compel formal, normative commitments to action. The achievement of such commitments has been signified by organizational changes such as developing EA-centered policy positions and policy statements; enacting relevant laws, resolutions, or standard operating procedures; creating units officially dedicated to and charged with addressing the problem; and fashioning specialty tracks, concentration areas, or curricula to instill/ensure applicable competencies.

The third and final goal of framing EA as a public health problem has been to provide necessary information so that appropriate decisions can be made about the appropriate level of resources needed to address EA. The use of this frame alongside frames of EA as an aging issue, as a crime, and as a human rights violation has increased substantially since the late 1990s. Increasingly, more stakeholders have adopted all-encompassing frames or alternated between different frames to help inform different constituencies and decision makers so that they may respond appropriately to address EA. These strategies have been used to help inform decisions that will support EA initiatives to levels and mixtures that are commensurate with the scale, complexity, and dynamics of this problem. The incorporation of the public health frame into the mix of strategies previously employed helped shift the discourse away from the perception of EA as a problem to be handled principally by one or two sectors and toward a perspective that addressing EA requires resources from multiple sectors because it involves and impacts multiple dimensions of health and social life, as argued earlier in this chapter.

ELDER ABUSE IS THE PUBLIC'S HEALTH PROBLEM

EA is more than just a public health problem: It is also the public's health problem. This specific framing of EA is essential, as it is a problem that the American public thinks about only in very abstract terms and experiences only episodically in a largely detached way (Volmert & Lindland, 2016). EA only occasionally becomes concrete, real, and fully present in the eyes of the public. When the confluence of specific events and incidents is brought to the forefront of society by news outlets and other media venues. Even on the rare occasions when this problem breaches the public's consciousness (e.g., Mickey Rooney, Brooke Astor), its impacts are fleeting and superficial because its significance to and implications for the life of the average person are perceived as low or unrelatable. The salience of EA is even more attenuated because the public may not regard it as an ominous problem or may consider it a problem that is less threatening than other problems that society must confront (i.e., it is a problem that impacts distant others). Consequently, even though segments of the American public are aware of EA and its consequences for public health, heretofore there has been little incentive for the public as a whole to make it a priority for societal action.

A report released by the FrameWorks Institute and focused on the gaps between expert and public understandings of EA in America indicates that the public does not see EA as its own issue and devotes little attention to it (Volmert & Lindland, 2016). The public's ambivalence and indifference regarding EA may be problematic because public motivation can lead to systemic actions to repel public health threats. In its absence, decision makers in critical sectors are less likely to understand EA as an urgent, important matter deserving of immediate attention and action and warranting the allocation of resources commensurate to eradicate the problem.

The framing of EA as the public's health problem is neither congruent with nor resonates with the personal, everyday experiences of individual members of the public body. Many individuals do not (think they) personally know someone who has experienced EA. Others may have observed problematic behaviors formally considered EA but have failed to recognize the behaviors as problematic generally or as abusive, neglectful, or exploitative specifically. Still others may consider the behaviors problematic and even abusive but chose to ignore, dismiss, or rationalize the behavior as isolated incidents. In each of the aforementioned situations, EA is interpreted as an unfortunate occurrence that is uncommon, extreme, or atypical. Sometimes, it is difficult to recognize or take signs of EA seriously. EA could appear to be symptoms of dementia or signs of an older adult's frailty—or caregivers may explain them as such. In fact, many of the signs and symptoms of EA do overlap with symptoms of mental deterioration (Robinson & Saisan, 2016). As a result, EA may not be afforded the appropriate recognition or response as a problem that the public is facing and must face collectively.

In reality, EA is a relatively common occurrence, involves problematic behaviors and experiences of variable severity, and can include single as well as repeated acts or failures to act. It is time that the public interest embraces ownership of this problem, given that EA is experienced by at least one out of every 10 older adults. Moreover, it is a problem with which each American must ostensibly contend, as most aging individuals eventually become older adults. Thus, among each group of 10 constructed from our older relatives, friends, neighbors, and acquaintances, at least one person may experience some form of abuse, neglect, or exploitation. Furthermore, as we ourselves become and live our lives as older adults, one out of every 10 of us may well face this problem. From this perspective, EA is not a distant or abstract threat, but rather a real and insidious threat to our personal well-being and to that of the older adults who matter to us the most. Also, the real and insidious threat of EA occurs precisely at a time in our lives when, individually, we may be the most powerless to ward off the problem.

The framing of EA presented here explicitly seeks to eliminate perceptions of this problem as a matter facing only older adults as a group that is often seen and discussed as somehow "different and separate" from other segments of America's population. Recognition of EA as a problem for the entire population of the United States—older adults as well as those who love and care for them—is critical to ensure that neither EA nor the plight of all those affected by it will be ignored.

Each member of the American public is morally compelled to work with and on behalf of older adults to create arrangements and environments that promote welfare, prevent harm, and eliminate and alleviate suffering when it occurs. Each time an elder is subjected to any of the adverse exposures and experiences associated with EA, individually and collectively, we should be disturbed, outraged, and compelled to take action. These reactions should create sustained institutional and societal changes to improve the present and future life conditions experienced in older adulthood.

Embracing EA as the public's health problem communicates and conveys the message that the lives, fates, and health states of older adults, younger adults, youth, and children are all inseparably intertwined and interdependent. Consequently, investments and actions to address EA will accomplish more than instituting changes that will benefit the older adult population alone. When combined with actions to reduce and prevent the forms of violence impacting other age groups, they will contribute to the creation of a nation where people of all ages and communities of all kinds are safer, healthier, and well positioned to enjoy prosperity and contribute to the public good.

ELDER ABUSE IS PUBLIC HEALTH'S PROBLEM

EA is also public health's problem. The introduction of this additional frame is necessary because public health has not, as a sector, assumed full ownership of EA as a problem with which it should and must deal. This present reality exists despite the fact that EA has clear implications for the public's health and for the operations of public health systems and agencies. Public health's reluctance to address EA may arise in part because many public health professionals do not themselves see or think of EA as a public health problem. Most undergraduate, graduate, and postgraduate public health trainings do not incorporate content, exposures, or experiences that provide specific insights into EA as a health topic or into EA prevention as a concentration for public health practice. In addition, work to address EA is not required of most state and local health departments to carry out essential public health services. In the absence of professional socialization that calls attention to and presents models for understanding and approaching this problem, many public health professionals may not be fully aware of EA's public health impacts or know how to use their training and skills to address it. Few public health agencies or organizations have the authority or the infrastructural capacity to implement EA-focused programs. Together, these conditions serve to reinforce the perception that addressing EA is not public health's responsibility.

Although the constraints created by the aforementioned conditions should not be minimized, it is important to consider why the problem of EA is and should be considered public health's problem or, more appropriately, public health's concern. The precedent for public health work in this domain is well established in several areas of public health practice. The most obvious of these precedents entails the specific focus of some members within the public health sphere on promotion of healthy aging. This particular objective and its supporting tasks were wisely embraced by public health decades ago, in light of and in response to observed and expected sociodemographic transitions, trends in the prevalence and impacts of chronic disease, and achievements in the extension of life expectancy.

Achievements in life expectancy were attained as public health and clinical medicine grew steadily more adept in dealing with and limiting the effects of infectious diseases and sources of unintentional injury. These health threats had historically set limits on the average life span of adults in the United States. Gains in preventive medicine and public health practice removed these constraints, allowing life expectancy to be extended by decades. These achievements paved the way for sociodemographic transitions that signaled the beginninng of a new era of older adulthood, where life could be lived to its fullest and society could continue to benefit from the presence and contributions of its oldest members.

Unfortunately, as the threats posed by acute conditions declined, their niche was filled by conditions and diseases whose course and impacts were of a more enduring nature. These emergent chronic threats to public health make a concentrated and increased focus on older adulthood essential. Although many of the factors associated with the onset of chronic diseases occur early in life, the diseases themselves and their sequelae tend to become more prevalent and/or severe with age.

As health leaders in society reflected on the health and demographic transitions occurring across the nation, it quickly became evident that the steady growth of the older adult population and the growing problem of chronic disease within this population could easily strain and outstrip the resources of public health, healthcare financing, and healthcare delivery systems (Goulding, Rogers, & Smith, 2003; Mrsnik, Beers, Morozov, & Standard and Poor's, 2010; Prince et al., 2015; World Health Organization & National Institute on Aging, 2011). It also became clear that the presence of chronic disease could create circumstances in which extensions in longevity would not necessarily be accompanied by increased or preserved quality of life during older adulthood. This eventuality could transform older adulthood into a period of life characterized by an increased disease burden, in which individuals would live longer but demonstrate far worse health states than previous generations. Public health evolved to face this challenge by developing units that would work directly to promote healthy aging. To this day, the sector retains components that actively identify, create, and enact policies and programs designed to promote, protect, and preserve the health and well-being of older adults and to ensure that health is maximized as the public ages.

From an operational standpoint, EA is public health's problem because it impedes progress toward ensuring optimal health in older adulthood. EA is itself a source of injuries, disabilities, and dysfunctions that compromise health, create functional impairments, and reduce quality of life. The individual and overlapping effects of different types of EA produce harms that endanger health in ways that are not typically addressed or accounted for by prevailing approaches to promoting healthy aging. Such approaches often focus primarily on early detection and prevention of diseases, rather than on the prevention of abuse, neglect, and exploitation. To achieve the conditions necessary for older adults to enjoy good health and well-being, it is essential that EA prevention be considered for inclusion in public health's agenda for promoting healthy aging, given its status as a fundamental cause of injury and poor health.

EA can also exacerbate the existing health conditions of those who experience it. This can occur most directly via physical damage or injuries to the body and its structures and systems. However, exacerbation can also occur indirectly by intensifying the anxiety and stress experienced by victims (which can, in turn, affect immune system functioning, cognitive status, and emotional stability) or by depleting or removing access to protective coping and social support resources (Begle et al., 2011; Luo & Waite, 2011; Wong & Waite, 2017). Through either of the pathways, EA interacts with and amplifies the health-related stressors already afflicting those exposed to it. Moreover, the complications and setbacks associated with EA may confound the provision of public health services by attenuating the effectiveness of health promotion actions taken by public health professionals.

Finally, EA can disrupt or prevent self-care, health promotion, and disease management activities. The coercive, controlling, and exploitive behaviors associated with some forms of EA can prevent individuals from completing activities necessary to maintain and improve their health (e.g., diet, exercise, foot care, and blood glucose testing among persons with diabetes).

These behaviors may also prevent older adults from accessing beneficial interactions specifically designed to decrease health risks or to promote management of existing health conditions (e.g., appointments with health-care providers such as physicians, optometrists, and counselors; preventive screening programs; immunizations; tai chi for falls prevention). It is through these additional impacts that EA further erodes the lives of older adults. Likewise, it is through such dynamics that EA can complicate and frustrate the work of the health promotion and disease/injury prevention specialists who serve older adults.

The work of public health professionals does not end with the provision of services to address the direct features and facets of the conditions of primary concern. The work of public health professionals also extends to ensuring the safety of those served, given the presence of factors or circumstances that may increase risks for victimization and other negative outcomes. Many conditions that become more common with age are accompanied by health-related vulnerabilities that may place older adults at increased risk for EA victimization. For example, some sources of cognitive impairment, such as dementia, stroke, and fall-related traumatic brain injuries, may increase victimization risks by reducing decision-making or disclosure abilities. In addition, visual impairments associated with cataracts, diabetes, hypertension, or hypercholesterolemia may impair self-protection capacities or abilities to effectively critique legal documents, such as contracts. To fully advance and safeguard client well-being, it is important for public health professionals working with older adults with such impairments to understand and work to address the EA-related risks these impairments introduce.

In the preceding paragraphs, EA was described as public health's problem, because its existence creates difficulties for those persons working in public health. The premise of this framing is that EA must be addressed because of its effects on public health's primary interests and its impacts on the sector's ability to perform its official duties. EA is more than just an obstacle, annoyance, or inconvenience—and public health can do more than simply "attend to" EA because it complicates other activities. Specifically, this sector can help evolve thinking about its causes and how it can be more proactively addressed.

Public health is part of an interdependent community of sectors that shares the task of promoting and protecting the public's welfare and well-being. Other sectors may be officially or more directly responsible for addressing EA. Distinct from other sectors, the public health sector can assist these sectors in fulfilling their responsibilities. Enhancements to EA prevention efforts resulting from public health's collaborative involvement confer collective benefits for all involved sectors. Most importantly, the populations targeted by these sectors may be better positioned to live safely and enjoy good health.

There are numerous ways in which public health can join other sectors in addressing EA. A hallmark of public health is that its toolkit includes a variety of specific alternatives for collaborative leadership and involvement, which are presented in depth in other chapters of this book. Two main opportunities for action are described here as this chapter's concluding act: (a) completing and strengthening the interpretive frames used to pursue EA-related action and (b) developing and enhancing capacities for the primary prevention of EA.

Completing and Strengthening Interpretive Frames for EA

At this point, it should be evident that interpretive frames have the potential to shape actions and efforts to address EA. They determine thoughts about the innate characteristics of the problem such as its characteristics and impacts. They may also influence ideas about its causes, solutions, and ownership.

Most existing EA frames are purely descriptive in nature. They describe the problem's character, scope, and consequences and may include statements about who in the society has a responsibility for addressing it (e.g., all Americans, everyone, and persons working in criminal justice). Few frames explicitly and strategically present information about what causes, contributes to, or affects the likelihood of EA. Even fewer propose specific effective or promising strategies for its prevention.

This tendency may be one reason why the prevailing frames often successfully generate general support for efforts to address EA, yet fail to elicit the precise types or levels of action desired by EA prevention stakeholders. In the absence of specifics regarding causes and possible solutions, public audiences and decision makers draw on default understandings and conceptions of EA that depict it as analogous to child abuse or domestic violence and that portray it largely as a criminal justice or Adult Protective Services issue. Using these frames as a reference point creates situations where EA may be accepted as a public health problem but continue to be primarily responded to as a crime. Such situations are undesirable because no new actions, or the wrong actions, may be taken to address the problem.

A second characteristic of existing frames for EA may also limit the field's success where the achievement of policy and practice actions is concerned—namely, the field has not reached broad consensus on what constitutes credible indicators. As is noted at several points throughout this book, there is no single, universally accepted estimate of either the prevalence or the incidence of EA. This lack of agreement arises because different data sources, methods, and approaches yield highly variable findings owing to differences in the purpose and scope of each data collection effort. Furthermore, although population-based prevalence studies have been conducted and provided informative snapshots of EA prevalence for specific periods, data of this type are not collected on an ongoing basis at local, state, or national levels. Given the variability in estimates of the magnitude of EA and the lack of data describing changes in its incidence and prevalence over time, decision makers may not have adequate information to make decisions about how to address this important issue.

The characteristics highlighted here, while problematic, also present public health with a unique opportunity to demonstrate its usefulness where the framing of EA is concerned. As a sector and a field of practice unto itself, public health is defined by specific analytic and methodological skill sets and concentrations of expertise that can be drawn on to help complete and strengthen existing interpretive frames used to seek action to address EA. First, public health's innate emphasis on risk and protective factors as an element of prevention can be modeled to simply and clearly describe those classes of factors that can be modified to decrease risks for EA perpetration and victimization. This could assist with presenting specific stakeholders with concrete, actionable "targets" for attention within strategies intended to address EA and its consequences. Second, specific effective or promising prevention or intervention strategies could be showcased within technical packages. Such packages, which have proved useful in promoting action to address other public health problems, offer specific directions for actions to achieve stakeholder goals, suggest approaches (e.g., programs, policies, or practices) that can be used to pursue these goals, and present the best available research evidence supporting the use of each described approach. Finally, public health's vast expertise in engaging stakeholders to achieve measurement standardization could be leveraged to promote data harmonization and reconciliation. This expertise could help achieve the desperately needed uniformity of "voice" needed to enhance the actual and perceived credibility of estimates of EA's magnitude and severity.

Developing and Enhancing Capacities for the Primary Prevention of EA

Most of the sectors traditionally viewed as responsible for addressing EA were designed to respond to this problem after perpetration has already occurred. In the aftermath of abusive experiences, these sectors treat harms inflicted upon individuals, act to limit the impacts of these adverse experiences, and take steps to stop further perpetration and/or reduce the likelihood of revictimization. Many of these sectors acknowledge the need to complement such reactive responses with more proactive strategies directed toward the primary prevention of EA (in which actions are taken to prevent the onset of EA). However, only a few of these sectors have acted to address EA as a health problem experienced by whole populations, and even fewer have adopted population-based, primary prevention–oriented approaches.

The broad acceptance of EA as a "public health problem" provides the public health sector with an opportunity to cultivate and extend a focus on the primary prevention of EA within the field. Public health can make the most of this opportunity by collaborating with professionals in other sectors to demonstrate and make the case that actions must be taken to prevent EA from ever occurring. This could be done by building upon existing research about the factors influencing the likelihood of EA to develop and by systematically testing and assessing the effectiveness of EA prevention policies, programs, and practices. This might also involve efforts to highlight and spread the word about existing primary prevention–oriented programs whose effectiveness and pathways of effect have been established or whose effectiveness requires further examination to fully characterize their utility. Finally, public health could work with other sectors to systematically document the best practices and procedures for implementing strategies and approaches for the primary prevention of EA. Special attention could be given to establishing the relationships, resources, and infrastructures required to achieve population-level impacts using the examined strategies.

SUMMARY

This chapter describes EA in three distinct, yet interrelated contexts of perception, interpretation, and action. In each context, a unique argument is made for acknowledgment, acceptance, and ownership of this problem. In reality, EA encompasses all three aspects. It is more than just an individual concern; the scope of its impacts and consequences and the harms visited on society make it a true public health problem. Moreover, EA is not just a problem facing and affecting older adults; its existence has implications for all individuals personally or professionally connected to older adults and for any person who hopes to live to a ripe "old age." Although EA may be addressed by other sectors, it affects the work of the public health sector and is a matter that public health has collective responsibility to address.

It is critical that EA be thought of in relation to each articulated interpretive frame as solutions for this problem are sought, considered, planned, and implemented. It is even more essential that such considerations and activities take place within—and with the assistance of—public health, given the potential facilitative role that this sector may play in advancing work to measure, monitor, and address EA more systematically and robustly at a population level. Public health's scientific and practice-related "powers" and capacities must be used for the good of older adults and, by extension, for the public good of the entire U.S. populace. We, the authors, challenge public health professionals at every level of operation to thoughtfully consider and embrace the ways of working suggested in this chapter. We hope that what we have written here will be extended as the reader considers and consumes each subsequent chapter, and that the provided content will promote and facilitate action by those who are the heads, hands, and hearts of public health.

REFERENCES

Acierno, R., Hernandez, M. A., Amstadter, A. B., Resnick, H. S., Steve, K., Muzzy, W., & Kilpatrick, D. G. (2010). Prevalence and correlates of emotional, physical, sexual, and financial abuse and potential neglect in the United States: The National Elder Mistreatment Study. *American Journal of Public Health, 100*(2), 292–297. doi:10.2105/ajph.2009.163089

Aravanis, S. C. (2002). *The National Policy Summit on Elder Abuse.* Binghamton, NY: Haworth Maltreatment & Trauma Press.

Begle, A. M., Strachan, M., Cisler, J. M., Amstadter, A. B., Hernandez, M., & Acierno, R. (2011). Elder mistreatment and emotional symptoms among older adults in a largely rural population: The South Carolina elder mistreatment study. *Journal of Interpersonal Violence, 26*(11), 2321–2332. doi:10.1177/0886260510383037

Bonnie, R. J, & Wallace, R. B. (Eds.). (2003). *Elder mistreatment: Abuse, neglect, and exploitation in an aging America.* Washington, DC: National Academies Press.

Connolly, M., Brandl, B., & Breckman, R. (2014). *The elder justice roadmap: A stakeholder initiative to respond to an emerging health, justice, financial and social crisis.* Washington, DC: Department of Justice. Retrieved from https://www.justice.gov/file/852856/download

Dong, X., & Simon, M. A. (2011). Enhancing national policy and programs to address elder abuse. *Journal of the American Medical Association, 305*(23), 2460–2461. doi:10.1001/jama.2011.835

Dong, X., Simon, M., Mendes de Leon, C., Fulmer, T., Beck, T., Hebert, L., . . . Evans, D. (2009). Elder self-neglect and abuse and mortality risk in a community-dwelling population. *Journal of the American Medical Association, 302*(5), 517–526. doi:10.1001/jama.2009.1109

Goulding, M. R., Rogers, M. E., & Smith, S. M. (2003). Public health and aging: Trends in aging—United States and worldwide. *Journal of the American Medical Association, 289*(11), 1371–1373. doi:10.1001/jama.289.11.1371

Hall, J. E., Karch, D. L., & Crosby, A. E. (2016). *Elder abuse surveillance: Uniform d efinitions and recommended core data elements, version 1.0.* Atlanta, GA: Centers for Disease Control and Prevention, National Center for Injury Prevention and Control.

Institute of Medicine & National Research Council. (2014). *Elder abuse and its prevention: Workshop summary.* Washington, DC: National Academies Press.

Institute of Medicine Staff. 1988. *Future of Public Health.* Washington, DC: National Academies Press. doi:10.17226/1091

Lifespan of Greater Rochester, Inc., Weill Cornell Medical Center of Cornell University, & New York City Department for the Aging. (2011). *Under the radar: New York State Elder Abuse Prevalence Study.* New York, NY: Author.

Luo, Y., & Waite, L. J. (2011). Mistreatment and psychological well-being among older adults: Exploring the role of psychosocial resources and deficits. *Journals of Gerontology. Series B, Psychological Sciences and Social Sciences, 66*(2), 217–229. doi:10.1093/geronb/gbq096

MetLife Mature Market Institute, National Committee for Prevention of Elder Abuse, & Virginia Polytechnic Institute and State University. (2011). *The MetLife study of elder financial abuse: Crimes of occasion, desperation, and predation against America's elders.* Westport, CT: MetLife Mature Market Institute. Retrieved from https://www.metlife.com/assets/cao/mmi/publications/studies/2011/mmi -elder-financial-abuse.pdf

Mrsnik, M., Beers, D. T., Morozov, I., & Standard and Poor's. (2010). *Global Aging 2010: An irreversible truth.* Retrieved from www.ebrd.com/documents/ cse/pension-systems-global-aging.pdf

Ortman, J. M., Victoria A. Velkoff, V. A., & Hogan, H. (2014). *An aging nation: the older population in the United States.* (Current Population Reports: Population Estimates and Projections P25-1140). Retrieved from https://www.census.gov/ content/dam/Census/library/publications/2014/demo/p25-1140.pdf

Prince, M. J., Wu, F., Guo, Y., Gutierrez Robledo, L. M., O'Donnell, M., Sullivan, R., & Yusuf, S. (2015). The burden of disease in older people and implications for health policy and practice. *Lancet, 385*(9967), 549–562. doi:10.1016/S0140-6736(14)61347-7

Ramsey-Klawsnik, H., & Heisler, C. (2014). Polyvictimization in later life. *Victimization of the Elderly & Disabled, 17*(1), 3–6.

Robinson, L., Saisan, J. & Segal, J. (2016). *Elder Abuse & Neglect: Warning Signs, Risk Factors, Prevention, and Reporting Abuse.* Retrieved from https://www .helpguide.org/articles/abuse/elder-abuse-and-neglect.htm

University of Michigan Center of Excellence in Public Health Workforce Studies. (2013). *Public Health Workforce Enumeration, 2012*. Ann Arbor: Author.

U.S. Census Bureau, Population Division. (2015). Annual estimates of the resident population by single year of age and sex for the United States, States, and Puerto Rico Commonwealth: April 1, 2010 to July 1, 2014. Retrieved from https://factfinder.census.gov/faces/tableservices/jsf/pages/productview .xhtml?src=bkmk

Volmert, A., & Lindland, E. (2016). *"You only pray that somebody would step in": Mapping the gaps between expert and public understandings of elder abuse in America*. Washington, DC: FrameWorks Institute.

Wong, J. S., & Waite, L. J. (2017). Elder mistreatment predicts later physical and psychological health: Results from a national longitudinal study. *Journal of Elder Abuse & Neglect, 29*(1), 15–42. doi:10.1080/08946566.2016.1235521

World Health Organization. (2002). Abuse of the elderly. In E. G. Krug, L. L. Dahlberg, J. A. Mercy, A. B. Zwi, & R. Lozano (Eds.), *World report on violence and health* (pp. 123–146). Geneva, Switzerland: Author. Retrieved from http://www.who .int/violence_injury_prevention/violence/global_campaign/en/chap5.pdf

World Health Organization & National Institute on Aging. (2011). Global health and aging. Retrieved from http://www.who.int/ageing/publications/global_ health.pdf.

2

ELDER ABUSE AND THE CORE FUNCTION OF PUBLIC HEALTH: USING THE 10 ESSENTIAL PUBLIC HEALTH SERVICES AS A FRAMEWORK FOR ADDRESSING ELDER ABUSE

Shalon M. Irving* and Jeffrey E. Hall

Public health professionals interact with older adults in various contexts. As the U.S. population aged 65 years and older grows to an estimated 83.7 million by 2050, public health systems may be increasingly confronted with issues relevant to the protection of older adults and the prevention of elder abuse (EA). Multiple definitions of EA exist with varying levels of specificity; however, in an attempt to provide standardization, the Centers for Disease Control and Prevention (CDC) recently released a document outlining the uniform definitions and recommended data elements for public health surveillance related to EA. CDC defines EA as "an intentional act or failure to act by a caregiver or another person in a relationship involving an expectation of trust that causes or creates a risk of harm to an older adult" (Hall, Karch, & Crosby, 2016)—with "an older adult" typically being defined as a person aged 60 years or older based on the age cutoff used in the Older Americans Act (see Older Americans Act of 1965 [2006], Title 1—Declaration of Objectives; Definitions, Section 102.(a)(40)). Central to this definition are

---

Disclaimer: The findings and conclusions in this chapter are those of the authors and do not necessarily represent the official position of the Centers for Disease Control and Prevention.

* This chapter is dedicated to the memory of its lead author, Shalon Irving, PhD, MPH, MS, CHES, who passed away during the development of this book. Dr. Irving was both respected and appreciated for her intelligence, charisma, and passionate personality. Her efforts to promote elder abuse prevention as a public health priority represent a mere fraction of her intellectual life and professional legacy.

the intentionality of the act and the violation of the trust that is expected within the context of the relationship. The latter differentiates EA from more general forms of violence committed against older adults in the community setting (e.g., robbery, assault).

EA is not an isolated occurrence or one that is restricted to certain racial/ethnic groups or social classes, but rather represents a viable threat to all older adults—a subpopulation that experiences increased vulnerability to this specific form of interpersonal violence in part because of the effects of natural and pathological physical, mental, and social changes that become more prevalent with age (Baker, 2007; Peguero & Lauck, 2008). EA may occur in settings such as an older adult's own home (or that of relatives, friends, or caregivers), board and care homes, assisted living facilities, or nursing homes. and may occur as older adults move between these different contexts (Desmarais & Reeves, 2007). In fact, an estimated one in 10 community-dwelling adults (i.e., those living independently or with a family member) aged 60 years and older has experienced EA (Connolly & Trilling, 2014). According to Mosqueda, Burnight, Liao, and Kemp (2004), the increased mortality experienced by older adults who experience abuse and mistreatment requires both public and professional attention.

ELDER ABUSE AS A PUBLIC HEALTH CONCERN

In the United States, EA was first recognized as a social problem during the 1960s (Dyer, Heisler, Hill, & Kim, 2005; Koenig & DeGuerre, 2005; Moskowitz, 1998; Nerenberg, 2008; Payne & Berg, 2003; Quinn & Zielke, 2005; Teaster, Wangmo, & Anetzberger, 2010; Wolf, 1999). Most of the early work defined EA from the conceptual, research, and practice frameworks undergirding and embraced by aging services, criminal justice, and domestic violence prevention systems and networks (Nerenberg, 2008). Because the overall approach taken by the domestic violence sector is one focused on secondary and tertiary prevention of intimate partner violence (IPV) among women of reproductive age, EA has not been well integrated into prevention strategies (Otto & Quinn, 2007). As a result, addressing EA is largely considered the responsibility of social services, aging, or law enforcement agencies (Ehrlich & Anetzberger, 1991; Morgan, Johnson, & Sigler, 2006). For many years, only the departments, units, and agencies at local, state, and federal operational levels of these systems were recognized as having legitimate authority to address EA. Among them, Adult Protective Service (APS) emerged as a primary contributor in the response to EA in the United States. In addition to linking victims to direct services, APS provides guidance for methods of reporting and investigating suspected EA as well as information about who is required to report suspected abuse (i.e., mandatory reporters). These mandates, however, are state specific. Thus, although APS serves an important role in addressing EA, its structure and function are not inherently supportive of a systematic, integrated, or coordinated response at a national level.

The view that EA is a crime—and therefore primarily a problem for criminal justice to address—is directly linked to how efforts to address its occurrence are shaped. Framing EA as a crime that threatens the autonomy and rights of frail older adults in community settings (and possibly indicates some level of family dysfunction) directs attention to the abusive act itself and its consequences, yet fails to address the many antecedents and determinants or the implications and costs for communities, thereby reducing the likelihood that attention and resources will be directed at primary prevention of EA. Historically, the resources (e.g., personnel, services, infrastructures) to mitigate the consequences of EA have been those available in the arena of criminal justice (e.g., punishment) or medical and social services (e.g., treatment). More recently, however, there has been recognition of the need for inputs and insights not included in these sectors.

Although the recognition of EA as an issue worthy of prevention efforts emerged 40 to 50 years ago, the adoption of EA as a public health and safety issue addressable by federal public health leadership has occurred only in the past two decades. Specifically, in 2001, the National Policy Summit on Elder Abuse was convened by the National Center for Elder Abuse (NCEA), whose constituent partner agencies included the American Bar Association (ABA) Commission on Legal Problems of the Elderly, the Clearinghouse on Abuse and Neglect of the Elderly (CANE) of the University of Delaware, the National Association of Adult Protective Services Administrators (NAAPSA), the National Association of State Units on Aging (NASUA), the National Committee for the Prevention of Elder Abuse (NCPEA), and the San Francisco Consortium for Elder Abuse Prevention of the Institute on Aging (IOA). At the summit, the deliberations of 80 EA prevention experts from multiple disciplines and sectors within seven working groups produced 10 recommendations promoting a coordinated federal response to EA and proposing a national EA policy agenda (Aravanis, 2002; Nerenberg, 2002; United States Administration on Aging, National Association of State Units on Aging, & National Center on Elder Abuse, 2001). The first recommendation was to develop and implement a sustained national strategic communications program to educate the public on EA. The first noted component of this program involved encouraging the CDC to recognize EA as a public health issue.

PUBLIC HEALTH AS A FRAMEWORK

On both national and international levels, EA has been recognized as a human rights violation that threatens societal efforts toward healthy aging (Ingram, 2003). Although public health has not been a traditional partner in eliminating EA, its increasing contribution to the ongoing discourse about EA is grounded in an understanding that violence committed against elders is a preventable threat to health and well-being that must be addressed in a systematic manner. EA is a threat to collective and social health and requires exploration of community-level intervention and prevention efforts. Among the individual consequences of EA are its physical, psychological, and financial costs.

Numerous physical consequences of EA have been documented in the literature. The most commonly cited are welts, wounds, and injuries (bruises, lacerations, dental problems, head injuries, broken bones, pressure sores). Other documented physical impacts include nutrition and hydration issues, sleep disturbances, increased susceptibility to new illnesses (e.g., sexually transmitted diseases), recurrence or worsening of preexisting health conditions, and increased risks for premature death (Bonnie & Wallace, 2003; Davis, 2007; National Center on Elder Abuse, 2001; Wolf, 1997; Wolf, Daichman, & Bennett, 2002). Among individuals with no documented disability, EA is predictive of later disability, and is associated with increased utilization of healthcare services (e.g., emergency departments and hospitalizations; Anetzberger, 2004; Dong et al., 2009; Lachs, Williams, O'Brien, Pillemer, & Charlson, 1998; Lindbloom, Brandt, Hough, & Meadows, 2007).

In addition to the physical impacts, the established psychological consequences of EA include higher levels of psychological distress, emotional symptoms, and depression among elders who report experiences of EA (American Medical Association, 1990; Comijs, Penninx, Knipscheer, & van Tilburg, 1999; Corso, Mercy, Simon, Finkelstein, & Miller, 2007; Dong, 2005; Dyer, Pavlik, Murphy, & Hyman, 2000; Pillemer & Prescott, 1989; Spencer, 1999). Other forms of psychological impacts have been proposed as deserving of additional inquiry and are just beginning to be explored. Among these are increased risks for developing posttraumatic stress syndrome and other fear or anxiety reactions compared to other persons with histories of trauma and/or neglect, including younger populations.

The social consequences of EA may further restrict the ability of victims to access social services and networks to prevent subsequent EA or reduce its impacts. These include increased social isolation (because of self-withdrawal or perpetrator imposition) and often decreased social resources (social identities, supports, roles in key networks). The direct medical costs of injuries caused by EA are estimated to contribute more than $5.3 billion to the United States' annual health expenditures (Heisler, 2000; MetLife Mature Market Institute, National Committee for the Prevention of Elder Abuse, & Center for Gerontology at Virginia Polytechnic Institute and State University, 2009), whereas financial abuse by itself costs older Americans more than $2.9 billion annually (Collins, 2006; Lachs & Pillemer, 2004). These financial costs may also be due to increased expenditures on services to compensate for resources lost through exploitation and to identify and treat or rehabilitate EA victims (Mouton et al., 2004; National Center on Elder Abuse, 2001). Because EA contributes directly to the societal burdens of violence and injury of older adults, there is a common and growing interest in addressing the public health need.

To prevent EA, it is necessary to move away from the use of a medical model—the traditional approach to diagnosing and treating conditions, diseases, and illness predominantly practiced by Western physicians, where the focus is on physical or biological defects or dysfunctions within patients (O'Toole, 2013). On its own, this model is inefficient in addressing EA (Ingram, 2003). According to Lachs and Pillemer (2004), using a medical or clinical model is difficult in the case of EA because some older adults are brought to the healthcare setting by their abuser and, therefore, have a limited ability to disclose their victimization. Moreover, because there is no widely agreed-upon test or screening tool for forms of domestic violence such as EA, the medical approach is largely unable to detect and, in turn, respond to the contextual nuances of EA.

The mission and tools of public health work alongside and complement the strengths of other sectors in society that have historically worked to stop EA. Using a public health model provides important frameworks and conceptual approaches that position the field of public health well to make essential contributions to EA prevention. Specifically, public health is not meant to replace what is done, but rather to extend and enhance those components that already work well.

This chapter highlights EA as a preventable, public health problem and explores successes, issues, and challenges encountered in attempting to effectively address EA from a public health perspective. By linking the 10 essential public health services with other existing frameworks used in the fields of public health and violence, the chapter sets out a systematic and integrated approach to EA that can be actualized by public health practitioners at the federal, state, and local levels.

The 10 Essential Services of Public Health

Attempts to address EA as a public health concern may benefit greatly from the application of the 10 essential public health services that are associated with the three core functions of public health—assessment, policy development, and assurance. These 10 essential services describe how public health performs its basic responsibilities to (a) prevent epidemics and the spread of disease, (b) protect against environmental hazards, (c) prevent injuries, (d) promote and encourage healthy behaviors, (e) respond to disasters and assist communities in recovery, and (f) ensure the quality and accessibility of health services (for detailed discussions of the orientation and development of the 10 essential services, see American Public Health Association, 1998; Harrell & Baker, 1994; Public Health Functions Steering Committee, 1994). Public health is especially well positioned to make essential contributions to EA prevention (Institute of Medicine, 2002) because of its responsibilities and capacities for assessment (e.g., collecting, analyzing, and disseminating information), policy development (e.g., helping to formulate comprehensive public policies based on sound scientific knowledge), and assurance (e.g., providing the programs and services necessary to improve well-being [Baker & Koplan, 2002; Nakanishi, Nakashima, & Honda, 2010]). The 10 essential public health services are summarized here:

1. Monitoring health status to identify and solve community health problems

2. Diagnosing and investigating health problems and health hazards in the community

3. Informing, educating, and empowering people about health issues

4. Mobilizing community partnerships to identify and solve health problems

5. Developing policies and plans that support individual and community health efforts

6. Enforcing laws and regulations that protect health and ensure safety

7. Linking people to needed personal health services and assuring the provision of healthcare when otherwise unavailable

8. Assuring a competent public and personal healthcare workforce

9. Evaluating the effectiveness, accessibility, and quality of personal and population-based health services

10. Conducting research to obtain new insights and innovative solutions to health problems

Each of these areas of service and an initial set of thoughts on how it might be approached in relation to the prevention of EA is described in the following sections.

ESSENTIAL SERVICE 1: Monitoring Health Status to Identify and Solve Community Health Problems

To effectively address the problem of EA, or any public health problem, accurate estimates of the magnitude of the problem are needed. Public health surveillance and monitoring activities help us to better understand the prevalence and potentially the incidence of EA in our society and to observe how patterns in these measures are changing over time. Given the sensitive nature of EA and barriers to victims' reporting of such abuse (e.g., isolation, fear of retaliation, lack of knowledge about available services), it is not advisable to rely solely on administrative or official statistics (e.g., from police reports). Not surprisingly, Connolly and Trilling (2014) suggest that for every case of EA that is identified, there are as many as 23 unreported and unidentified victims. Thus, monitoring necessitates the incorporation of other approaches to estimate the burden of EA in society. There are laws in place that require the collection of data on EA; however, unlike for child abuse, systems to collect data on EA have not been widely established or implemented (Connolly & Trilling, 2014). Using the strengths of public health will help develop and coordinate new and/or enhance existing data systems to conduct EA surveillance across multiple sectors in the field. In the meantime, steps can be taken to explicitly train community-level workers (e.g., meals on wheels volunteers, home health service delivery personnel) to identify factors that might place older adults at greater risk of victimization. This may give them the ability to take steps to lessen the level of risk faced by the target populations whom they serve. In addition, this training should equip community-level workers with the knowledge of what abuse may look like and what its indications may be. Those individuals who have frequent contacts with older adults may further benefit from education on how to assist older adults in accessing services or on understanding EA reporting systems. Given that universal screening for EA has yet to be implemented because of lack of resources and the absence of a tool that could be easily and effectively used by a wide variety of sentinels, these other measures may capture data on those elders who participate in some community- or home-based services but are kept away from medical professionals either through self-isolation or restrictions imposed by an abuser. In addition, such measures may identify persons whose medical encounters may be limited because of mobility or transportation challenges, persons not requiring formal medical care because they are relatively healthy despite experiencing EA, and persons experiencing forms of EA for which medical care may not be sought (e.g., emotional, psychological, or financial EA).

Methodological and practical issues arise because of gaps or inconsistencies in conceptual understandings and operationalizations of EA. Lack of consistency in the terms used to describe EA may lead to miscommunication and difficulty forming partnerships and collaborations to address the problem (Otto & Quinn, 2007). The use of jargon often reinforces perceptions of differences between sectors and accentuates what may appear to be incompatible goals and interest. Moreover, sector-specific theories or models of EA may share many common elements but contain enough diversity to generate measures of EA that do not capture precisely the same aspects of EA. Such communication and measurement differences must be reconciled to allow coordinated use of existing EA data and to improve possibilities for data harmonization across sectors. Another point of inconsistency noted in EA prevalence studies conducted by researchers in a wide variety of fields involves the use of varying lower age thresholds to determine that an individual is classified as an older adult (Desmarais & Reeves, 2007). The sampling frames constructed using these different inclusion criteria will cover and exclude different populations. As a result, any prevalence estimates obtained from samples utilized will not be generalizable and may be pushed upward or downward depending on where the lower limit of older adulthood is placed (e.g., consider the number of additional possible cases that will be included when using an age threshold of 50 years and older versus an age threshold of 60, 65, or 70 years of age).

One example of how such challenges might be addressed using the strengths and public health surveillance expertise of public health is provided by the work of CDC. In 2016, CDC, in collaboration with a diverse group of experts from a variety of sectors in the field of EA prevention, released "Elder Abuse Surveillance: Uniform Definitions and Recommended Core Data Elements." This document has the potential to help standardize the collection of data relevant to EA locally and nationally and to "address data collection features that cause important discrepancies, gaps, and limitations in what is known about EA" (Hall et al., 2016). It was developed to help EA prevention stakeholders take more effective action to prevent and stop EA.

For example, local-level public health leaders might bring together different EA stakeholders to initiate or improve the monitoring of EA at local and state levels by promoting the collection of data using a public health surveillance framework. Frontline personnel interacting with personnel from other sectors could take steps to learn more about the specific data or reporting requirements that their colleagues or contemporaries in other sectors must meet and how such requirements affect the specific approach taken to how EA is identified, contextualized, and documented. They might also identify gaps in existing data sources and then identify appropriate data collection activities to address such gaps. Persons supervising frontline public health staff could ensure that frontline public health personnel have the necessary knowledge, skills, and abilities in the implementation of public health surveillance, as this area relates to the collection of data on EA. This might entail identification of opportunities to learn more about the considerations and challenges that distinguish EA surveillance from the public health surveillance conducted for other conditions affecting older adults. Finally, upper-level or senior managers might establish relationships, agreements, and infrastructures that could support more fluid data sharing across departments and agencies and/or create new possibilities for combining or pooling resources as part of collecting, analyzing, and applying EA data.

ESSENTIAL SERVICE 2: Diagnosing and Investigating Health Problems and Health Hazards in the Community

Diagnosing and investigating EA as a public health problem can help to better elucidate determinants, "comorbidities" or co-occurring factors, risk factors, and protective factors. Without knowledge of these factors, it is difficult to identify appropriate interventions (Bonnie & Wallace, 2003). According to Lachs and Pillemer (2004), collective understanding of the independent and shared risk factors for EA victimization and perpetration is still emerging. Therefore, carrying out ongoing epidemiologic analyses to continuously improve the field's understanding and knowledge of the relationships among the factors that influence the likelihood of EA is vital.

Public health researchers may examine interconnections among perpetration and victimization and how the dynamics of EA are not only influenced by the characteristics of the individuals involved in abusive interactions but also affected by relationship characteristics and features of larger social environments within the families, communities, and settings where abuse may occur. This work might also benefit from determining whether modifications of community-level variables aimed at lowering or reducing the likelihood of other forms of violence such as IPV or youth violence may also alter risks for the perpetration of EA. It is essential to better understand how experiences of EA are shaped and either permitted or precluded by social structures, so that actions to alter such structures can be devised and implemented to achieve EA prevention on a grander scale. Finally, in situations where data suggest that EA levels may be increasing or decreasing, public health personnel may be able to assist with investigations to identify the factors responsible for these changes and determine how the observed effects may have been achieved.

Initiatives to improve the effectiveness of risk assessment, case identification, and abuse investigations are also areas where public health expertise may prove useful. Public health has a long history of collaboration to develop and continuously refine tools and tactics for risk identification as well as screening for the presence of specific conditions or experiences, including violence and abuse. Such knowledge and expertise may prove essential as public health continues to examine the state of science as it relates to the screening for IPV and abuse of elderly and vulnerable adults. The most recent update of the U.S. Preventive Services Task Force analysis concluded that the current evidence is insufficient to assess the balance of benefits and harms of screening all elderly or vulnerable adults (physically or mentally dysfunctional) for abuse and neglect. This finding suggests a continuing need for information that can conclusively characterize the benefits of screening activities and provide leads regarding effective approaches and tools for their implementation (U.S. Preventive Services Task Force, 2013). Because it relates to risk assessment and case identification, special attention should be paid to how cognitively intact and impaired older adults are identified as having been victims of EA (McMullen, Schwartz, Yaffee, & Beach, 2014). Attention must be paid to the nuances of identification for these two very different groups, and public health's cognitive health–related insights regarding investigative tactics and the conditions under which data may be collected from groups with varying levels of cognitive capacity might prove valuable and timely.

The functions associated with diagnosis and investigation are at the core of what public health does best. Health departments and other public health organizations at the federal, state, and local levels are poised to perform these functions when resources are available to them. Resource needs include an appropriately trained workforce (see Essential Service 8), established systems of reporting and communication, and access to good-quality data—or the infrastructure through which to capture these data (Davis & Lederberg, 2000).

ESSENTIAL SERVICE 3: Informing, Educating, and Empowering People About Health Issues

Building knowledge and raising awareness about EA can help achieve the essential functions of public health to inform, people in regard to this health issue. This could include provision of content, materials, and communications that promote broad recognition of linkages among the numerous individual, relationship, family, and community characteristics that may influence risks for EA. Moreover, it could include sharing and making available information about evidence-based policies, programs, practices, and resources that might be adopted or adapted for local use in addressing EA. If the public does not understand what constitutes EA, what its signs and symptoms are, and how to prevent its occurrence and help victims, many cases of EA will go unreported and opportunities for interventions will be missed.

Although most efforts to inform, focus on older adults and the practitioners and providers who work with older adults, Podnieks and Thomas (2014) suggest that this process should begin much earlier in the life course and should include instilling in children positive images of older adults. Information and education campaigns that focus on a more mature population could consider multiple media for disseminating the messages, including social media (e.g., Twitter), health education, and health promotion campaigns. Such campaigns could be complemented with the development and provision of demographic, epidemiologic, scientific, and programmatic presentations for specific audiences and stakeholders to deepen familiarity with and appreciation of the nature and scope of EA. This form of understanding could support action to address EA that is more closely aligned with the specific needs present in communities, cities, and states, which could translate into aggregate protective benefits for older adults at the national level. Moreover, health education and health promotion partnerships could be developed or leveraged at local levels within communities and neighborhoods to help create structures designed to prevent or significantly reduce the likelihood of EA. Such partnerships may facilitate the provision of the most current information to individuals, families, and communities about how to prevent, recognize, stop, and recover after experiences of EA. They may also help create environments that overtly discourage abusive, neglectful, or abusive behavior.

By ensuring that information related to EA is distributed widely to older adults who may be experiencing neglect, to those who are not, and to the general population, the overall understanding of EA may continue to grow. As a result of education and information, these groups may feel more empowered, thereby creating a paradigm in which more and more persons and groups may be mobilized to quickly and effectively assist with its prevention. Public health agencies and systems could routinely provide infrastructure support for dissemination efforts to ensure that information about EA, alongside or in combination with other information, is distributed to older adults and to those interested in the well-being of older adults to promote healthy aging. Raising awareness about our societal investment in the safety and dignity of older adults is a widely embraced moral commitment (National Research Council, 2003).

Given that great cultural variability exists in the treatment of elders across groups, approaches directed toward education and empowerment related to EA and when to seek help for it (or report suspected abuse) may benefit from being culturally relevant. Because cultures have their own conceptualizations of what is acceptable regarding the treatment of elders, the norms and laws that prevail in society should be communicated so that all people, regardless of culture, know when a line has been crossed from the perspective of the larger U.S. society (Jervis, 2014). Nurturing of skills in recognizing, considering, and acting appropriately to account for the role of cultural and social factors may help shape audience receptivity to specific messages regarding EA.

ESSENTIAL SERVICE 4: Mobilizing Community Partnerships to Identify and Solve Health Problems

In the early 1980s and 1990s, the multidisciplinary approach to EA used a grassroots approach to organize community leaders in areas traditionally responsible for preventing and stopping EA. These leaders included researchers, practitioners, and activists (Podnieks & Thomas 2014). Now, effective multidisciplinary approaches require integration across an extensive variety of sectors and disciplines, including both those traditionally tasked with addressing EA (e.g., criminal justice and APS) and those less traditionally looked to as partners (e.g., businesses, faith-based organizations, anchor institutions) in these efforts (Ingram, 2003), in addition to policy makers and academics.

Public health has a tradition of integrative leadership through which a broad array of professions, organizations, and sectors work together to promote health and well-being, thereby responding to the public health clarion call for multisectoral and community partnerships (Frieden, 2014). Through these multisectoral collaborations, public health has successfully created clear case definitions for use in surveillance of illnesses, diseases, and injuries. This approach reduces the chance for duplication of services, centralizes prevention efforts, and leverages resources across sectors. To fully realize their potential to provide this essential service, these partnerships and collaborations must be collaboratively constructed to be fully transparent and accountable, because this will make it easier for other entities and agencies to understand how they may fit into efforts to address EA (Thomas, 2004).

Meaningfully engaging community-based organizations and other community-informed stakeholder groups in the development of approaches to address and reduce EA may help increasing cultural relevance of the solutions while also increasing the awareness of cultural issues among the public health practitioners. According to the U.S. Census Bureau, the composition of the older adult population is expected to become more diverse in the coming decades, with demographic changes including a dramatic increase in the number of racial and ethnic minority elders. Thomas (2004) recommends engagement of the community in conducting needs assessments, determining research priorities, and developing prevention efforts for EA. Even with the best available evidence of cultural differences between groups and the best-intentioned practitioners, without community input the interventions and prevention strategies proposed are likely to miss the mark. This is especially true among underserved and marginalized populations.

Public health expertise in areas such as community engagement and community-based participatory research could be drawn upon to create effective partnership arrangements and structures. Initially, such partnerships should be overtly goal based and focused on achievement of EA-related prevention and intervention objectives that are specific, measurable, achievable, realistic, and time bound, as such an orientation is associated with a greater likelihood of success within partnerships. They should also be constructed in ways that clearly specify the unique roles of each contributor as well as directly state and acknowledge acceptance of expectations governing interactions within the formed partnerships. Finally, the partnerships should include routines that ensure sufficient attention to issues such as sustainability and adequate resourcing over time. This final element is critical to ensure coalitions, and partnerships continue to contain the appropriate mixtures of members/partners, resources, and social capital required for optimal pursuit of EA prevention and intervention objectives.

Public health can also help to expand thinking about the many options for participation in partnerships focused on the problem of EA. The provision of funding resources to support activities is just one of several ways partners may add value to a mix of contributors. Another way to participate in a community partnership is through the provision of technical assistance (TA). When organizations and agencies possess subject matter or methodological expertise in a particular area, the science may best be advanced by helping partners with fewer resources conceptualize or design intervention/prevention projects or address definitional issues or issues requiring cultural competence or pertaining to cultural relevance. Other organizations recruited as partners may assist with gathering, accessing, analyzing, or interpreting data or community input to assure that policies, programs, and practices identified for use in addressing EA will have the characteristics associated with effective action (for information about the principles of effective programs, see Nation et al., 2003). Finally, public health personnel, particularly those in higher leadership levels, can play important facilitative roles in establishing linkages with key stakeholders who may not currently participate in partnerships or who are missing from planned partnerships. They may also, in some circumstances, help address and resolve relationship challenges that may complicate interactions among specific stakeholders, such as territorial conflicts between or within different sectors interacting with older adults.

ESSENTIAL SERVICE 5: Developing Policies and Plans That Support Individual and Community Health Efforts

In 2010, the Elder Justice Act (EJA; S.2933)—a comprehensive federal law addressing EA—was enacted (for a brief synopsis written by the Congressional Research Service, see www.govtrack.us/congress/bills/107/s2933/summary). To date, this law has not been fully implemented because of limited allocations of funding (Connolly & Trilling 2014). Although the passage of the EJA could be a useful policy step to help prevent EA, other gaps may still exist or become evident, particularly as population demographics shift.

Organizational policies may be needed to support efforts to improve health. However, on a larger scale, federal, state, or local policies can help to shape efforts and create opportunities for EA prevention. Public health has expertise in the evaluation of laws, policies, and legislation as it relates to conditions that affect public health. This expertise could be tapped to determine the advantages and disadvantages of proposed data collection and service provision methods and to identify examples or instances of effective functional policy and legislative options that could be examined for potential replication in different settings. Public health might also play roles in acquiring the three types of evidence that can help to comprehensively characterize the effectiveness of policies, programs, or practices enacted—contextual evidence, experiential evidence, and the best available research evidence (for more information about the three types of evidence, see Puddy & Wilkins, 2011). Once compiled, this store of evidence could be provided to the appropriate stakeholders for consideration and integration in decision making.

ESSENTIAL SERVICE 6: Enforcing Laws and Regulations That Protect Health and Ensure Safety

Mandatory reporting laws, which also depend on selected definitions, are established to protect vulnerable members of our society. Commonly associated with child abuse, mandatory reporting laws also endeavor to protect other individuals with increased vulnerability to abuse and neglect, such as people with disabilities and older adults. These laws ensure that some public-sector workers and health services professionals (e.g., teachers, doctors) and other individuals such as bankers, beauticians, and barbers who come in regular contact with vulnerable individuals are trained to recognize and report signs of abuse. In addition to children, people with disabilities and older adults are subpopulations covered under mandatory reporting laws—on the basis of their increased vulnerability to experiencing abuse and neglect.

Currently, the laws related to mandatory reporting differ by state. Recommendations made in 2001 by a panel of experts suggest not only that mandatory reporting laws should be the same nationally, but also that education and training should be provided so that mandatory reporters understand their mandate, what constitutes abuse, and the penalties for failure to report (Ingram, 2003). One criticism of EA mandatory reporting laws is that they are based on a child abuse model and so remove some degree of choice from cognitively intact elders who have a right to choose whether to report abuse and/or leave an abusive situation (Desmarais & Reeves, 2007). Public health professionals could help obtain more evidence regarding the true effectiveness of these laws (as well as other relevant legal authorities, statutes, codes, and regulations) and assist in clarifying the conditions, structures, and supports needed to optimize their effectiveness once implemented.

In addition, it is necessary to identify and assess the impacts of existing public health authorities, laws, or statutes addressing EA or EA prevention efforts. Nursing homes and other institutional settings could be more regularly assessed to determine whether they are in compliance with applicable laws, regulations, and ordinances. One way to address this may be to establish or enhance collaborations with long-term care ombudsmen to take actions necessary to ensure that regulations and laws governing such facilities are regularly reviewed and consistently enforced. Such efforts may help strengthen areas where reinforcement is lacking and inform policy development in situations where notable gaps are identified. Such collaborations may be particularly vital as new institutions emerge to effectively and judiciously address the needs of older adults with various health conditions requiring various levels of professional assistance.

In addition, enforcement activities may benefit from specific data and information about the contexts in which existing policies do not function as intended. Data regarding the moderators of policy effectiveness may help inform decisions about options to create environments where EA is less likely to occur, and actions that can be taken to ensure the feasibility of elected options in light of contextual factors (e.g., staffing levels relative to caseloads, particularly for services or sectors that may be needed to respond to the risk or presence of EA; availability of services tailored to the specific needs of subgroups within the older adult population, such as older adults who identify as lesbian, gay, bisexual, transgender, and questioning (LGBTQ); levels of technological sophistication; nature of the legal relations that exist among operatives in various sectors).

Public health personnel could also take steps to ensure that programs to promote and protect older adult are set up in ways that do not expose older adults to increased risk for abuse or exploitation. This is a particularly important consideration with programs that provide older adults with resources and assistance to cover basic needs, such as housing, food, and healthcare. These programs must be conceived and implemented in ways that guarantee that the benefits are enjoyed by their intended recipients and the opportunities for coercion, misuse, misappropriation, and exploitation are minimized. Those participating in program development, implementation, and evaluation can work actively to incorporate programmatic safeguards that increase the likelihood that the interests of older adults will be protected.

The Public Health Code of Ethics, which was developed to explicitly clarify the distinctive elements of public health and the ethical principles that follow from or respond to these elements (Thomas, Sage, Dillenberg, & Guillory, 2002), delves into how to accomplish each of the tasks associated with public health efforts in an ethical manner (Thomas, 2004). This issue is particularly important when addressing EA because it is a problem that may easily infringe on an individual's rights and, while not unethical, may not always rise to the level where formal or legal action is required.

ESSENTIAL SERVICE 7: Linking People to Needed Personal Health Services and Assuring the Provision of Healthcare When Otherwise Unavailable

Efforts to link and coordinate the provision of personal, social, and health services used by the various parties that may be involved in EA are critical. Such services may include primary prevention activities and programs that could reduce risks for victimization accessed either by older adults themselves or by persons and parties concerned with protecting the well-being of their older loved ones. In addition, secondary prevention or intervention-oriented services may be designed either to detect and stop abuse or to prevent revictimization among persons with a prior history of EA victimization. Finally, needed services might include initiatives or programs that can halt, limit, or reasonably manage the long-term physical, psychological, and social impacts upon and consequences of EA victimization for the lives of older adults and promote a return to normalcy after EA has ceased.

Two components of service provision are especially important to consider—the linking functions of public health service availability and service access. Although the availability of the three types of services outlined earlier is important and necessary to provide opportunities for the pursuit of optimal health in the face of EA, persons and groups that may consume and use such services must also be aware of their existence, aware that they qualify for them, and able to access them without fear of repercussion. If any of these three conditions is not present, then older adults and other important constituencies may not receive exposures, contacts, or resources that could prevent or stop EA or limit its associated health impacts. Multi-sectoral partnerships can help explore the ability of nontraditional partners to make community-based referrals to personal, social, and health services when EA victimization or perpetration is possible, suspected, or confirmed (see Chapter 6).

It is necessary to consider engagement strategies to identify and then link socially isolated victims to services. As stated earlier, social isolation is a risk factor for victimization among older adults (Lachs & Pillemer, 2004). The nature of the relationship is complicated because some EA victims self-isolate, whereas others are isolated by their abusers through force, coercion, or both. Regardless of the nature of social isolation, it prevents older adults from accessing or receiving needed services. This may especially be true if healthcare professionals such as medical doctors or healthcare interactions within community public health services are the only instances where referrals for services are possible.

Because older adults may have limited support resources (because of the deaths of spouses, friends, and other loved ones), they may have difficulty identifying alternatives to remaining in abusive situations (Otto & Quinn, 2007). These older adults may choose to remain in abusive environments rather than risk institutionalization. Although unlikely to be a primary solution, support groups can often help to provide needed social support, thereby reducing social isolation, reminding older adults that many of their experiences are shared with their peers, and providing a venue for the dissemination and acquisition of information and education materials that may assist older adults in taking steps to escape or stop EA.

It may occasionally be useful for public health personnel to help inform policies and protocols that focus on service referral, care coordination, and information-sharing activities. This process may also help create and provide resources for initiatives to remove access barriers to vital services and eliminate systemic "holes" that allow persons with significant needs/problems to "disappear" or their problems to go undetected.

ESSENTIAL SERVICE 8: Assuring a Competent Public and Personal Healthcare Workforce

According to Ingram (2003), "training for practitioners is critically important in all disciplines associated with efforts to stem the tide of elder mistreatment" (p. 62). Across numerous disciplines, there appears to be a shortage of competent, adequately trained public health workers who are poised to address EA (Connolly & Trilling, 2014).

One way that public health personnel in managerial and supervisory positions can take steps to assure the development of a competent public and personal care workforce is to collaboratively identify the specific educational and training needs of the public health workforce with regard to this problem. This can be accomplished in a number of ways, including conducting system-level needs assessments; identifying general violence prevention and EA-specific competency domains for which knowledge, skills, and abilities must be instilled and cultivated; and examining public health pedagogical and professional socialization structures for points where new training and educational opportunities are negotiated and subsequently integrated. Identified competencies should align different levels of professional practice, including frontline staff, senior level staff, and supervisory or management staff, consistent with the approaches used by groups such as the Council on Linkages Between Academic and Public Health Practice.

Moreover, explicit efforts are needed to create academic partnerships to promote development of public health professionals with knowledge of and skills in geriatrics, gerontology, and other disciplines playing vital roles in promoting healthy aging. In doing so, academic programs (and other partners) should be appropriately engaged as collaborators to ensure that the future workforce possesses subject matter-specific knowledge and recognizes how to conduct work that is culturally sensitive and ethical. Such actions could, in turn, be followed with efforts to create workforce and individual development plans including training, exercises, immersive experiences, and communities of practice to instill and continuously refresh skills in violence prevention as it relates to EA. This should include active efforts to seek, identify, or create opportunities for individual, team/unit, and organizational learning and development focused on EA as well as efforts to establish mentoring, peer advising, coaching, or other personal development opportunities to deepen prevention-related skills and expertise.

As a final step, practice tools and guidelines are necessary to govern EA assessment, detection, and intervention activities. Such tools and guidelines could help structure and inform decision making and action aimed at providing older adults with services that can prevent or stop abuse and ensure fidelity in the implementation of prevention activities and programs.

ESSENTIAL SERVICE 9: Evaluating the Effectiveness, Accessibility, and Quality of Personal and Population-Based Health Services

Process, outcome, and impact evaluation processes must be built into prevention or intervention efforts. Plans for evaluation should be clearly outlined and explicitly include a strategy for integrating information received from a mixture of sources to improve current efforts in real time and to show how changes in outcomes are to be achieved and identified as distinctly attributable to the actions implemented (rather than deriving from other extraneous historical or contextual influences). Sufficient steps to document activity implementation should provide critical lessons learned to inform future actions to improve and extend EA prevention efforts. It is important to cultivate professional cultures and partnership arrangements conducive to and supportive of conducting systematic, scientifically rigorous evaluations that will clearly establish what works to prevent EA, as well as the efficacy of specific activities.

It is important to pursue evaluations (especially evaluations of effectiveness) when they have not been done in this setting, even if the approach is not new. Indeed, public health builds assessment into one of its core competencies. It is critical to use the best and most appropriate evaluation methods and measures to ensure that public health accomplishes this lofty goal.

ESSENTIAL SERVICE 10: Conducting Research to Obtain New Insights and Innovative Solutions to Health Problems

Although the first nine essential services focus primarily on practice and policy, the 10th essential service hones in on related research needs. The development of policies aimed at primary prevention can be hindered by a lack of data. Connolly and Trilling (2014) note that five areas need improvement to address what they call egregious gaps hindering policy development: intervention, defining success, prevention, data collection, and cost.

An especially important research domain to which public health stands to contribute pertains to factors influencing population-based risks for EA. Our understanding of risk factors must be dynamic and flexible because older adults are a highly diverse population. Research is required to further clarify whether the contributions of some factors to risks for EA are more potent than others (and if so, which factors exhibit these effects and what might happen to population health if their effects could be removed or reduced); how the odds, extent, and pattern of EA change when more of these factors are present; and whether specific combinations of factors heighten or significantly reduce vulnerability to EA. Finally, mediating and moderating relationships that explain how or why certain factors influence risks for EA should be investigated.

Practitioners should be trained and supported to develop rigorous evaluations of existing and newly conceived EA and other violence- or injury-prevention programs. It is essential to focus on identifying effective and promising approaches to EA prevention to measurably reduce the prevalence of EA. Evaluation research will help clarify prevention activities that work, if they are replicable, and in which settings. Findings have the potential to inform policies, programs, or practices for implementation on a broader scale at state or national levels. Identifying and monitoring innovative solutions and cutting-edge research are, therefore, vitally necessary to advance public health efforts to protect and preserve older adults' health via EA prevention.

THE ROAD AHEAD

Framing action using the 10 essential public health services charts a course for public health personnel so that they can contribute to existing efforts to address EA. Moreover, the methods, approaches, and strengths of public health are a formidable foundation from which interdisciplinary relationships can be forged to strategically pool, combine, and better leverage resources to support the elimination of EA. Such partnerships may be well positioned to address issues and challenges that have stymied progress in protecting both the older adult population as a whole and specific subsegments of it. The cross-fertilization of diverse insights and expertise may yield innovative, new solutions.

For example, one challenge confronting EA professionals involves determining which kind or type of approach to address EA is most useful when dealing with cognitively intact older adults who decide to stay in environments that are violent or neglectful (Mosqueda et al., 2004). Even though the underlying philosophy is that abuse of older adults is wrong and should be prevented or eliminated, unlike children, cognitively intact older adults have a right to make what others might regard as deleterious decisions. Public health professionals specializing in public health ethics could work closely with ethicists in other coordinating sectors to research, develop, and evaluate the trade-offs in costs versus benefits of specific strategies aimed at assisting this population. These novel strategies may be distinctly different from the traditional approaches to EA, such as developing a safety plan (Lachs & Pillemer, 2004). However, they may also offer new opportunities for realizing policy and practice achievements that have long proved elusive.

The first step toward a more meaningful integration of public health principles, practices, and persons in work to address EA must occur within public health itself. Public health as a sector, practice area, and science must become more familiar with the problem of EA and better acquainted with and open to the possible options for involvement to prevent and stop its occurrence. This chapter has provided and described just a small selection of such options related to existing services implemented within public health to promote and protect population health generally and among older adults specifically. The provided examples could stimulate additional thinking about other ways that public health and its numerous agents might contribute to and add value to efforts already under way in other sectors that have been traditionally responsible for handling the problem of EA.

Thinking about public health's inherent talents and native ways of serving the population generally, and older adults specifically, is a necessary action to increase the possibility of leveraging public health's strengths and functions in ways that can create the safe, stable, and nurturing relationships and environments that can effectively prevent older adults from experiencing EA. We challenge others in the field of public health to thoughtfully consider ways that EA might be incorporated into their scope of work. We argue that public health is poised to use what we know and what we do well to create prevention-centered arrangements, initiatives, and resources to increase opportunities for everyone to experience older adulthood as a period of life forever free from abuse, neglect, and exploitation.

REFERENCES

American Medical Association. (1990). American Medical Association white paper on elderly health: Report of the Council on Scientific Affairs. *Archives of Internal Medicine, 150*, 2459–2472. doi:10.1001/archinte.1990.00390230019004

American Public Health Association. (1998). *The essential services of public health.* Washington, DC: Author.

Anetzberger, G. (2004). *The clinical management of elder abuse.* New York, NY: Hawthorne Press.

Aravanis, S. C. (2002). *The National Policy Summit on Elder Abuse.* Binghamton, NY. Haworth Maltreatment & Trauma Press.

Baker, E. L., Jr., & Koplan, J. P. (2002). Strengthening the nation's public health infrastructure: Historic challenge, unprecedented opportunity. *Health Affairs, 21*(6), 15–27. doi:10.1377/hlthaff.21.6.15

Baker, M. W. (2007). Elder mistreatment: Risk, vulnerability, and early mortality. *Journal of the American Psychiatric Nurses Association, 12*(6), 313–321. doi:10.1177/1078390306297519

Bonnie, R. J., & Wallace, R. B. (Eds.). (2003). *Elder mistreatment: Abuse, neglect, and exploitation in an aging America.* Washington, DC: National Academies Press.

Collins, K. A. (2006). Elder maltreatment: A review. *Archives of Pathology & Laboratory Medicine, 130*(9), 1290–1296. Retrieved from http://www.archivesofpathology.org/doi/full/10.1043/1543-2165%282006%29130%5B1290%3AEMAR%5D2.0.CO%3B2?code=coap-site

Comijs, H. C., Penninx, B. W., Knipscheer, K. P., & van Tilburg, W. (1999). Psychological distress in victims of elder mistreatment: The effects of social support and coping. *Journals of Gerontology, Series B: Psychological Sciences and Social Sciences, 54*(4), P240–P245. doi:10.1093/geronb/54B.4.P240

Connolly, M. T., & Trilling, A. (2014). Seven policy priorities for an enhanced public health response to elder abuse. In Institute of Medicine & National Research Council (Eds.), *Elder abuse and its prevention: Workshop summary* (pp. 59–66). Washington, DC: National Academies Press.

Corso, P. S., Mercy, J. A., Simon, T. R., Finkelstein, E. A., & Miller, T. R. (2007). Medical costs and productivity losses due to interpersonal and self-directed violence in the United States. *American Journal of Preventive Medicine, 32,* 474–482. doi:10.1016/j.amepre.2007.02.010

Davis, J. R., & Lederberg, J. (Eds.). (2000). Public health systems and emerging infections: Assessing the capabilities of the public and private sectors (Workshop summary). Retrieved from http://www.nap.edu/catalog/9869.html

Davis, R. C. (2007). *Victims of crime.* Thousand Oaks, CA: Sage.

Desmarais, S. L., & Reeves, K. A. (2007). Gray, black, and blue: The state of research and intervention for intimate partner abuse among elders. *Behavioral Science & the Law, 25,* 377–391. doi:10.1002/bsl.763

Dong, X. (2005). Medical implications of elder abuse and neglect. *Clinics in Geriatric Medicine, 21*(2), 293–313. doi:10.1016/j.cger.2004.10.006

Dong, X., Simon, M., Mendes de Leon, C., Fulmer, T., Beck, T., Hebert, L., ... Evans, D. (2009). Elder self-neglect and abuse and mortality risk in a community-dwelling population. *Journal of the American Medical Association, 302*(5), 517–526. doi:10.1001/jama.2009.1109

Dyer, C. B., Heisler, C. J., Hill, C. A., & Kim, L. C. (2005). Community approaches to elder abuse. *Clinics in Geriatric Medicine, 21*(2), 429–447. doi:10.1016/j.cger.2004.10.007

Dyer, C. B., Pavlik, V. N., Murphy, K. P., & Hyman, D. J. (2000). The high prevalence of depression and dementia in elder abuse or neglect. *Journal of the American Geriatrics Society, 48*(2), 205–208. doi:10.1111/j.1532-5415.2000.tb03913.x

Ehrlich, P., & Anetzberger, G. (1991). Survey of state public health departments on procedures for reporting elder abuse. *Public Health Reports, 106*(2), Retrieved from http://www.ncbi.nlm.nih.gov/pmc/articles/PMC1580213

Frieden, T. R. (2014). Six components necessary for effective public health program implementation. *American Journal of Public Health, 104*(1), 17–22. doi:10.2105/AJPH.2013.301608

Hall, J., Karch, D., & Crosby, A. (2016). *Elder abuse surveillance: Uniform definitions and recommended core data elements for use in elder abuse surveillance, version 1.0.* Atlanta, GA: National Center for Injury Prevention and Control, Centers for Disease Control and Prevention.

Harrell, J. A., & Baker, E. L. (1994). The essential services of public health. *Leadership in Public Health, 3*(3), 27–31.

Heisler, C. J. (2000). Elder abuse and the criminal justice system: New awareness, new responses. *Generations: The Journal of the Western Gerontological Society, 24,* 52–58.

Ingram, E. M. (2003). Expert panel recommendations on elder mistreatment using a public health framework. *Journal of Elder Abuse & Neglect, 15*(2), 45–65. doi:10.1300/J084v15n02_03

Institute of Medicine. (2002). *The future of the public's health in the twenty-first century.* Washington, DC: National Academies Press.

Jervis, L. L. (2014). Native elder mistreatment. In Institute of Medicine & National Research Council (Eds.), *Elder abuse and its prevention: Workshop summary* (pp. 75–79). Washington, DC: National Academies Press.

Koenig, R. J., & DeGuerre, C. R. (2005). The legal and governmental response to domestic elder abuse. *Clinics in Geriatric Medicine, 21*(2), 383–398. doi:10.1016/j.cger.2004.11.001

Lachs, M. S., & Pillemer, K. (2004). Elder abuse. *Lancet, 364,* 1263–1272. doi:10.1016/S0140-6736(04)17144-4

Lachs, M. S., Williams, C. S., O'Brien, S., Pillemer, K. A., & Charlson, M. E. (1998). The mortality of elder mistreatment. *Journal of the American Medical Association, 280*(5), 428–432. doi:10.1001/jama.280.5.428

Lindbloom, E. J., Brandt, J., Hough, L. D., & Meadows, S. E. (2007). Elder mistreatment in the nursing home: A systematic review. *Journal of the American Medical Directors Association, 8*(9), 610–616. doi:10.1016/j.jamda.2007.09.001

McMullen, T., Schwartz, K., Yaffee, M., & Beach, S. (2014). Elder abuse and its prevention: Screening and detection. In Institute of Medicine & National Research Council (Eds.), *Elder abuse and its prevention: Workshop summary* (pp. 88–94). Washington, DC: National Academies Press.

MetLife Mature Market Institute, National Committee for the Prevention of Elder Abuse, & Center for Gerontology at Virginia Polytechnic Institute and State University. (2009). *Broken trust: Elders, family & finances.*Westport, CT: Authors. Retrieved from http://www.gerontology.vt.edu/docs/mmi-studies-broken-trust.pdf

Morgan, E., Johnson, I., & Sigler, R. (2006). Public definitions and endorsement of the criminalization of elder abuse. *Journal of criminal justice, 34*(3), 275–283.

Moskowitz, S. (1998). Saving granny from the wolf: Elder abuse and neglect: The legal framework. *Connecticut Law Review, 31,* 77–201.

Mosqueda, L., Burnight, K., Liao, S., & Kemp, B. (2004). Advancing the field of elder mistreatment: A new model for integration of social and medical services. *Gerontologist, 44*(5), 703–708. doi:10.1093/geront/44.5.703

Mouton, C. P., Rodabough, R. J., Rovi, S. L., Hunt, J. L., Talamantes, M. A., Brzyski, R. G., & Burge, S. K. (2004). Prevalence and 3-year incidence of abuse among postmenopausal women. *American Journal of Public Health, 94*(4), 605–612. Retrieved from https://ajph.aphapublications.org/doi/full/10.2105/AJPH.94.4.605

Nakanishi, M., Nakashima, T., & Honda, T. (2010). Disparities in systems development for elder abuse prevention among municipalities in Japan: Implications for strategies to help municipalities develop community systems. *Social Science & Medicine, 71*(2), 400–404. doi:10.1016/j.socscimed.2010.03.046

Nation, M., Crusto, C., Wandersman, A., Kumpfer, K. L. Seybolt, D., Morrissey-Kane, E., & Davino, K. (2003). What works in prevention: Principles of effective prevention programs. *American Psychologist, 58*(6–7), 449–456. doi:10.1037/0003-066X.58.6-7.449

National Center on Elder Abuse. (2001). *Proceedings of the National Policy Summit on Elder Abuse: Creating the action agenda*. Washington, DC: The National Association of State Units on Aging.

Nerenberg, L. (2002). The National Policy Summit issue briefs. *Journal of Elder Abuse & Neglect, 14*(4), 71–104. doi:10.1300/J084v14n04_07

Nerenberg, L. (2008). *Elder abuse prevention: Emerging trends and promising strategies*. New York, NY: Springer Publishing.

Older Americans Act of 1965. Pub. L. 89–73, 70 Stat. 218 (2006). Retrieved from https://legcounsel.house.gov/Comps/Older%20Americans%20Act%20Of%201965.pdf

O'Toole, M. T. (2013). *Mosby's medical dictionary* (9th ed.). St. Louis, MO: Elsevier/ Mosby.

Otto, J. M. & Quinn, K. (2007). *Barriers to and promising practices for collaboration between Adult Protective Services and domestic violence programs: A report for the National Center on Elder Abuse*. Retrieved from http://www.californiamenscenters .org/wordpress/wp-content/uploads/2009/04/barriers-to-collaborationaps -and-dv-programs.pdf.

Payne, B. K., & Berg, B. L. (2003). Perceptions about the criminalization of elder abuse among police chiefs and ombudsmen. *Crime & Delinquency, 49*(3), 439–459. doi:10.1177/0011128703049003005

Peguero, A. A., & Lauck, A. M. (2008). Older adults and their vulnerabilities to the exposure of violence. *Sociology Compass, 2*(1), 62–73. doi:10.1111/j.1751 -9020.2007.00055.x

Pillemer, K., & Prescott, D. (1989). Psychological effects of elder abuse: A research note. *Journal of Elder Abuse and Neglect, 1*(1), 65–73. doi:10.1300/ J084v01n01_06

Podnieks, E., & Thomas, C. (2014). Preventing elder abuse: Hope springs eternal. In Institute of Medicine & National Research Council (Eds.), *Elder abuse and its prevention: Workshop summary* (pp. 75–79). Washington, DC: National Academies Press.

Public Health Functions Steering Committee. (1994). *Public health in America*. Washington, DC: Author.

Puddy, R. W., & Wilkins, N. (2011). *Understanding evidence part 1: Best available research evidence. A guide to the continuum of evidence of effectiveness*. Atlanta, GA: Centers for Disease Control and Prevention.

Quinn, K., & Zielke, H. (2005). Elder abuse, neglect, and exploitation: Policy issues. *Clinics in Geriatric Medicine, 21*(2), 449–457. doi:10.1016/j.cger .2005.01.002

Spencer, C. (1999). *Exploring the social and economic costs of abuse in later life*. Vancouver, Canada: Simon Fraser University.

Teaster, P. B., Wangmo, T., & Anetzberger, G. J. (2010). A glass half full: The dubious history of elder abuse policy. *Journal of Elder Abuse & Neglect, 22*(1–2), 6–15. doi:10.1080/08946560903436130

Thomas, J. (2004). *Skills for the ethical practice of public health.* Retrieved from https://nnphi.org/wp-content/uploads/2015/08/ph-code-of-ethics-skills-and -competencies-booklet.original.pdf

Thomas, J. C., Sage, M., Dillenberg, J., & Guillory, V. J. (2002). A code of ethics for public health. *American Journal of Public Health, 92*(7), 1057–1059. Retrieved from https://ajph.aphapublications.org/doi/full/10.2105/AJPH.92.7.1057

U.S. Preventive Services Task Force. (2013). Screening for intimate partner violence and abuse of elderly and vulnerable adults: U.S. Preventive Services Task Force recommendation statement. *Annals of Internal Medicine, 158*(6), 478–486. doi:10.7326/0003-4819-158-6-201303190-00588

Wolf, R. S. (1997). Elder abuse and neglect: Causes and consequences. *Journal of Geriatric Psychiatry, 30*(1), 153–174.

Wolf, R. S. (1999). Elder abuse. In V. B. Van Hasselt & M. Hersen (Eds.), *Handbook of psychological approaches with violent offenders: Contemporary strategies and issues* (pp. 373–393). New York, NY: Kluwer Academic/Plenum Press.

Wolf, R. S., Daichman, L., & Bennett, G. (2002). Abuse of the elderly. In E. G. Krug, L. L. Dahlberg, J. A. Mercy, A. B. Zwi, & R. Lozano (Eds.), *World report on violence and health* (pp. 123–146). Geneva, Switzerland: World Health Organization.

3

ELDER ABUSE AND THE ROLE OF PUBLIC HEALTH LAW AND HEALTH SERVICES ADMINISTRATION

Emmanuel D. Jadhav and James W. Holsinger, Jr.

Elder abuse (EA) is a complex situation, the prevalence and incidence of which is not fully known, and policy development is still in its early stages. Only in recent years has EA gained attention as a social problem that lacks policy and administrative direction. The purpose of this chapter is to identify the characteristics of EA from a public health administration perspective and to relate it to the types of abuse delineated by the National Center on Elder Abuse guidelines. The three core functions of public health services and the 10 essential public health services are introduced. The legal policies associated with elder care and the institution and administration of EA law through public health policies are discussed using the Commonwealth of Kentucky as a case study.

Chapter Objectives

By the end of this chapter, readers will be able to

1. Describe the three core public health functions and 10 essential public health services and their relationship to EA.

2. Describe legal policies associated with elder care and abuse.

3. Understand the scope of public health services administration and its impact on EA.

4. Understand how social legislation has impacted EA.

5. Describe why and how EA is a public health issue.

6. Understand how the framework of "prevalence, diagnosis, societal impact, and preventability" (PDSP) may be applied to identify public health issues.

Thinking about EA is likely to conjure up images of vulnerable elderly individuals with an unkempt appearance with bruising and scars telling their tale of being victims of spousal, family, and/or nursing home abuse or even street crime or fraud. This perception coincides with that observed by Rowe and Kahn in *Successful Aging*, in which they determined that elders are viewed as those individuals who are sick and frail, ranging from being demented, weak, disabled, powerless, sexless, passive, or alone to simply being unhappy (Rowe & Kahn, 1999). In Shakespeare's famous "Seven Stages of Man" speech in the play *As You Like It*, a somber Jacques describes the final stage of life as "second childishness and mere oblivion, sans teeth, sans eyes, sans taste, sans everything" like "the infant, mewling and puking in the nurse's arms" (Shakespeare, 2004). This state of childlike dependency in the later stages of life creates an imbalance in caregiving and care receiving roles. Although it is difficult to imagine a caregiver intentionally mistreating an elderly person or being unable to recognize that the person is being mistreated, it is plausible that in the transition from the traditional caregiver to the care receiver role, abuse may occur either intentionally or unintentionally. Thus, as a construct, abuse may occur intentionally; however, from a public health standpoint, abuse requires behavioral intentionality because of the public health focus on prevention. The etiologic contexts of intentional and unintentional injuries differ, as do the types of actions required to prevent and address them. Consequently, discussion of both the intentional and unintentional aspects of abuse is warranted.

When considering the health status of elderly individuals, a well-being continuum can be represented at the robustness/resilience pole by the Viagra-touting elder population exuding vigor and robust health, walking into the sunset holding hands and romantically gazing into each other's eyes. Thus, implying that the elder population is not entirely made up of persons on the weakness/frailty pole of the continuum, who are frail, weak, or disabled. Some studies have identified that purposeful living, access to nutritious food, safe exercising places, and affordable healthcare are some of the elements of healthy aging (Boyle, Barnes, Buchman, & Bennett, 2009; Rowe & Kahn, 1999). It is within this continuum of frail and weak elders and robust and vigorous elderly persons that mistreatment is found and gives newfound meaning to Clark's observation that "we've put more effort in helping folks reach old age than into helping them enjoy it" (Singh, 2005).

Although the extent of EA is not fully known, its social and moral significance is obvious. Given society's efforts to maintain privacy concerning personal matters such as the family, EA is a social problem that is often hidden from public view. However, evidence is accumulating that indicates EA is both an important public health problem and an important societal problem. Public health services administration is a key element for addressing EA.

DISCUSSION BOX

Rebecca is a retired high school math teacher from northwest Michigan. She is in her early 70s, has a valid driver's license, and occasionally drives herself around town. She is quite alert and cognizant for her 75 years of age. Rebecca was always known to be a fiercely independent woman, so it did not surprise her family and friends when she decided to continue staying in the family home after her husband of 55 years passed away.

Unfortunately, Rebecca suffered a bad fall at home and became bedridden. Other than being a bit confused at times, Rebecca appeared to handle the situation quite well. Her designated caregiver is her son, who lives 5 miles away. The son and daughter-in-law have jobs that take them outside the city during the day, so they check in on Rebecca in the mornings before heading to work for the day. They ensure that food and water are within easy reach for her. They have also hired home health nurses to visit her on alternating days. When they return in the evenings, they check on Rebecca to meet and attend to her needs. At night, Rebecca's granddaughter sleeps at Rebecca's home, providing care until she leaves for work at noon the next day.

With all this caregiving in place, her son is extremely surprised to receive a call from the community hospital. The physicians have ascertained that Rebecca is suffering from extreme dehydration and has lost significant weight since her fall. She also suffers from bladder and bowel incontinence and has a bed sore on her buttocks. The physician is unsure that her family is treating her properly, whereas the family believes that they are doing their very best to care for her.

The nation's public health system has a significant role to play in ensuring that a strong infrastructure is in place to enable elderly persons at all socioeconomic levels to exercise purposeful living, to have access to nutritious food, to enjoy safe places to exercise, and to obtain affordable healthcare. EA demands a multifaceted response that can be delivered through the complex public health delivery mechanisms that interact with third-party care providers to focus on protecting the right of older individuals to age safely (Paul, 2002). This chapter reviews the conceptual understanding of EA, introduces public health services administration, describes some of the legal policies associated with EA, and explains the interaction of public health services administration and public health law and policy to address EA, using the institution of Adult Protective Services (APS) in Kentucky as a case study.

ELDER ABUSE

Although historically elder mistreatment has been a private situation, the recognition of elder mistreatment's significance as a societal issue has been growing in recent decades (Fulmer & O'Malley, 1987). Deliberation about the issue is still subdued and emotionally charged because behaviors inside the home continue to be considered a private affair, even though the home has long been considered a place of security. Reports suggest that one in 10 older adults in the United States has experienced physical, psychological, or sexual abuse, neglect, or financial exploitation (Institute of Medicine, n.d.). Many of the victims are frail and vulnerable older individuals who cannot help themselves and depend on others to meet their most basic needs—a plausible explanation as to why EA is often unreported. Because caregivers are often family members, friends, or a "trusted other," the prevailing cultural norm of "home affairs remaining private acts" serves as a deterrent to reporting EA. Unfortunately, the failure to report EA is in keeping with the traditional American idea of home, and consequently it interferes with the recognition of and response to EA.

The Generational Inversion Rate

The high generational inversion rate—that is, the inversion of roles earlier held by the parent—is a significant issue when dealing with elder mistreatment (Steinmetz, 1988). Never before have so many middle-aged and young-old adult children (age 55–75 years) been required to care for elderly parents. This phenomenon can be attributed to advances in public health that have added 25 years to the average life span (Bunker, Frazier, & Mosteller, 1994) in conjunction with medical advances. The geriatric populace is the most rapidly growing age group in the United States, comprising 46 million in 2016 and expected to increase to more than 98 million by 2060. The 65 years and older age group's share of the total U.S. population is expected to increase from 15% to nearly 24% during the same period of time (Mather, Jacobsen, & Pollard, 2015). Individuals reaching age 65 years have an average life expectancy of an additional 19.2 years (20.4 years for females and 17.8 years for males). Older women outnumber older men by 24.3 million to 18.8 million. In 2013, 36% of older women were widows. Older men were much more likely to be married than older women—71% of men versus 45% of women. Approximately 28% (12.1 million) of noninstitutionalized older persons live alone (8.4 million women, 3.7 million men), with nearly half of women (45%) aged 75 years and older living alone. In 2012, approximately 518,000 grandparents aged 65 years or older had the primary responsibility for their grandchildren who lived with them.

Although one study found an incidence of one in 10 adults experiencing abuse, it did not include financial abuse (Teaster et al., 2004). The median income of older persons in 2012 was $27,612 for males and $16,040 for females, and approximately 9.1% were below the poverty level (Centers for Disease Conrol and Prevention, n.d.). These numbers are conservative estimates because they do not account for intentional changes in lifestyle behaviors that extend longevity.

The lack of a data repository concerning EA is a significant issue interfering with the progress of research and qualitative and quantitative studies of the issue; as well as with efforts to obtain public health resources for services to prevent, halt, and address EA. The National Elder Abuse Incidence Study, conducted more than a decade ago, was the first major investigation of abuse of elders in the United States; since then, data on EA have continued to be scattered and limited. The original National Elder Abuse Incidence Study found that approximately 500,000 persons aged 60 years or older had been physically abused, neglected, or in some way mistreated in 1996 (National Center on Elder Abuse & American Public Human Services Association, 1998). More recent studies have estimated the incidence of EA and neglect at 7.6% to 10% (Acierno et al., 2010; Lifespan of Greater Rochester, Weill Cornell Medical Center of Cornell University, & New York City Department for the Aging, 2011). Most cases of abuse, neglect, and exploitation go undetected and untreated, with one study estimating that only one in 14 cases of EA comes to the attention of the authorities (Bonnie & Wallace, 2003). The New York State Elder Abuse Prevalence Study found that for every case known to programs and agencies, 24 were unknown (Lifespan of Greater Rochester et al., 2011). Thus, the data confirm that each year, hundreds of thousands of older persons are abused, neglected, and exploited.

PUBLIC HEALTH PERSPECTIVE OF ELDER ABUSE

Public Health Administration and Elder Abuse

Public health administration includes the leadership, management, and administration of public health systems (Ferris State University, n.d.). In the United States, public health is practiced through the collective actions of governmental and private organizations that vary widely in their resources, missions, and operations (Halverson et al., 1996; Mays, Miller, & Halverson, 2000). The public health system comprises "all public, private, and voluntary entities that contribute to the delivery of essential public health services within a jurisdiction" (Centers for Disease Control and Prevention [CDC], 2007). Hospitals, public safety agencies, voluntary health organizations, mental health centers, schools, civic groups, faith institutions, and many others contribute to accomplishing the actions necessary to protect the public's health. However, governmental public health agencies are the leaders in the public health system and form its core at the federal, state, and local levels (Committee on Assuring the Health of the Public in the 21st Century, 2002). At the federal level, the Department of Health and Human Services (DHHS) is the primary agency for overseeing the health of Americans as well as providing individuals with essential public health services (U.S. DHHS, n.d.). Nongovernmental public health agencies include hospitals, universities, grassroots consumer organizations, national professional organizations, and other private-sector organizations (Institute of Medicine & Committee for the Study of the Future of Public Health, 1988).

Public health administration includes the leadership, management, and administration of all these agencies to improve the health and well-being of the population by virtue of its collective emphasis on preventive care. Thus, EA is within the service scope of public health agencies because prevention is associated with behavioral intentionality, which construes abuse. EA has been defined as "an intentional act or failure to act by a caregiver or another person in a relationship involving an expectation of trust that causes or creates a risk of harm to an older adult" (Hall, Karch, & Crosby, 2016). Elder maltreatment—a term used interchangeably with EA—refers to any knowing, intentional, or negligent act by a caregiver or any other person that causes harm or a serious risk of harm to a vulnerable older adult (AoA, n.d.; Quinn & Tomita, 1997).

The concept of intentionality in both these definitions merits a clear understanding of intentionality in the case of elder mistreatment. It is possible that the intent to cause damage may not be the primary motive of a caregiver, leading to differences between intentional behavior and consequences (World Health Organization, 2002). For example, the actions of the caregivers in the case study of Rebecca, while concerning to the physician, may not be perceived as negligent by the caregivers because there was probably no intent to harm Rebecca. Likewise, contextual understanding is important in determining intentionality. In some contexts, a power relationship that uses intimidation and force may not appear out of the ordinary. These behaviors, however, could be considered acts of abuse if they have important health consequences for the care-receiving elder. Using the example of Rebecca's case study, if the prevailing norm of the context in which she lives makes her son the decision maker for her treatment choices, and he refuses to invest her resources for her treatment, resulting in her poor health status, then his actions could be considered abusive in nature.

The missions of the various public health agencies are well aligned to assist with containing and controlling EA stemming from intentional violation of an older adult's fundamental right to well-being and to be safe and free from violence (Taylor, 2013). A 1988 Institute of Medicine (IOM) report, *The Future of Public Health*, describes the mission of public health as "fulfilling society's interest in assuring conditions in which people can be healthy" (Institute of Medicine & Committee for the Study of the Future of Public Health, 1988). The CDC, which is the nation's leading disease prevention and wellness promotion agency, defines public health as "the science of protecting and improving the health of families and communities through detection and control of infectious diseases, research for disease and injury prevention, and the promotion of healthy lifestyles." (CDC Foundation, n.d.). *The Dictionary of Public Health Promotion and Education* defines public health as "[p]reventing disease, prolonging life, and promoting health and efficiency through organized community efforts for the sanitation of the environment, control of communicable infections, education in personal hygiene, organization of medical and nursing services, and development of the social machinery to ensure everyone a standard of living adequate for the maintenance of health" (Modeste & Tamayose, 2004). The Association of Schools and Programs of Public Health (ASPPH) utilizes the CDC definition of Public Health. The common theme running through all of these definitions is captured in the World Health Organization's (WHO's) definition of public health as "the science and art of preventing disease, prolonging life, and promoting health through the organized efforts of society" (WHO, n.d.).

As discussed in greater detail in Chapter 2, "Elder Abuse and the Core Function of Public Health," attending to a nation's socioeconomic status and publichealth practices, such as education in environmental sanitation and personal hygiene, have a greater impact on the health of a population than all the biomedical interventions combined (Lee, 2012). Publication of the IOM's *The Future of Public Health* in 1988 drew renewed attention to public health, making it relevant to the modern era. This report set out three core functions of public health and also identified the 10 essential public health services to guide the management and administration of public health agencies (Table 3.1; Institute of Medicine & Committee for the Study of the Future of Public Health, 1988). The three core functions include assessment, policy development, and assurance.

Assessment: As part of this function, public health agencies are expected to regularly and systematically collect, assemble, analyze, and make available information about the health of the community, including statistics on health status, community health needs, and epidemiologic and other studies of health problems.

Policy development: Within this function, public health agencies are expected to participate in the development of comprehensive public health policies that are in the public's interest. Public health agencies are encouraged to promote the use of evidence-based decision making, implying that agencies would need to develop a strategic approach using the democratic political process.

Assurance: The third core function recommended by the IOM committee is for public health agencies to assure their constituents that services necessary to achieve mutually agreed community health goals are available. The expectation is that public health agencies will engage with community stakeholders and key policy makers to determine high-priority personal and community-specific health services that need to be guaranteed to every member of the community. This guarantee includes, but is not limited to, the subsidization or direct provision of high-priority personal health services

TABLE 3.1 THE 10 ESSENTIAL PUBLIC HEALTH SERVICES
1. Monitor health status to identify community health problems.
2. Diagnose and investigate health problems and health hazards in the community.
3. Inform, educate, and empower people about health issues.
4. Mobilize community partnerships to identify and solve health problems.
5. Develop policies and plans that support individual and community health efforts.
6. Enforce laws and regulations that protect health and ensure safety.
7. Link people to needed personal health services and assure the provision of healthcare when otherwise unavailable.
8. Assure a competent public health and personal healthcare workforce.
9. Evaluate the effectiveness, accessibility, and quality of personal and population-based health services.
10. Conduct research to obain new insights and innovative solutions to health problems

Source: Data from Institute of Medicine & Committee for the Study of the Future of Public Health. (1988). *The future of public health.* Washington, DC: National Academies Press.

for those unable to afford them (Institute of Medicine & Committee for the Study of the Future of Public Health, 1988).

On its surface, the relationship between controlling EA and public health administration appears straightforward, especially because the focus of public health intervention is on prevention through surveillance of cases and the promotion of healthy behaviors. Coupled with the advancements in technology and the professional responsibilities (Schmutzler & Holsinger, 2011) of healthcare providers, public health administration is very well positioned to assist with EA.

PUBLIC HEALTH LAW, PUBLIC HEALTH ADMINISTRATION, AND ELDER ABUSE

For public health administrators to provide the 10 essential public health services to elders and to provide assessment, policy development, and assurance in the protection of elders, public health law is of prime importance.

Public health law is the basis on which public health administrators provide services to not only elders, but also the population at large. The practice of public health administration is dependent on a broad array of legal sources, including the U.S. and state constitutions, legislative enactments, promulgated regulations, common law, and treaties. Public health law provides the basis for governmental power and duty to provide for and assure the conditions under which the health of the population, or a subset of the population such as elders, may be assured. It is the body of law that establishes an elder's right to live in a healthy environment (DeBuono & Tilson, 2003). Public health administration is specifically responsible for providing services to elders under three of the 10 essential public health services: Essential Service 5, Developing policies and plans that support individual and community health efforts; Essential Service 6, Enforcing laws and regulations that protect health and ensure safety; and Essential Service 9, Evaluating effectiveness, accessibility, and quality of personal and population-based health services.

To fully understand the responsibilities of public health administrators, a working definition of public health law is required. Public health law may be defined as

> . . . the study of the legal powers and duties of the state, in collaboration with its partners, to assure the conditions for people to be healthy (e.g., to identify, prevent, and ameliorate risks to health in the population) and the limitations on the power of the state to constrain the autonomy, privacy, liberty, proprietary, or other legally protected interests of individuals for the common good. The prime objective of public health law is to pursue the highest possible level of physical and mental health in the population, consistent with the value of social justice. (Gostin & Wiley, 2007)

This definition of public health law forms the basis for all public health administrative actions taken to preserve and protect the health and well-being of the elder population.

Goodman describes seven models that could be used to safeguard the health and well-being of elders and for the prevention of disease and injury (Table 3.2; Goodman et al., 2007). The power to tax and spend enables governmental units such as states and localities to provide the funds for ensuring the safety of elders in long-term care facilities as well providing the staff required to investigate EA. The power to alter the informational environment can protect elders not only by mandating appropriate labeling of pharmaceuticals, but also by providing the context within which APS

TABLE 3.2 PUBLIC HEALTH LAW MODELS TO SAFEGUARD THE HEALTH AND WELL-BEING OF ELDERS
Model 1: Power to tax and spend
Model 2: Power to alter the informational environment
Model 3: Power to alter the built environment
Model 4: Power to reduce socioeconomic disparities
Model 5: Direct regulation of individuals
Model 6: Indirect regulation through the tort system
Model 7: Deregulation

Source: Adapted from Goodman, R. A., Hoffman, R. E., Lopez, W., Matthews, G. W., Rothstein, M., & Foster, K. (Eds.). (2007). *Law in public health practice.* New York, NY: Oxford University Press.

may assist elders who are mistreated. The power to alter the built environment can be used to provide safe places for elders to engage in the activities of daily living. The power to reduce socioeconomic disparities provides a financial safety net for elders who do not possess the funds to maintain themselves at a healthy level. The direct regulation of individuals can be used to assist elders through the regulation of long-term care facilities as well as the licensing of healthcare practitioners. Likewise, this aspect of public health law may assist in protecting elders from being abused financially. Use of the tort system on behalf of the public's health can be used to assist elders who have been financially abused or physically harmed. Deregulation is useful to elders in that the constant review of the regulatory powers of government results in public health regulations meeting the current social environmental needs of elders.

Public health law is essential in establishing the three core functions in public health agencies. The three core functions (assessment, policy development, and assurance), although overlapping, encompass the full spectrum of public health administrative activities—from surveillance activities to determine the extent of EA, to development of policies to protect elders from abuse, to assurance that the services necessary to achieve high-priority personal and community-specific health services are available to protect elders from such actions on the part of others. Without the underpinnings provided by law and regulation, public health administrators would be unable to protect elders from abuse or to rectify injustices that have occurred.

Against the backdrop of the personal nature of EA, only recently has addressing EA as social policy moved to the forefront of public health law and policy development. The six federal agencies that have traditionally been involved in addressing EA through their programs and research are the National Institutes of Health (NIH), CDC, Administration on Community Living (ACL), Department of Justice's Civil Division, National Institute of Justice, and Office of Victims of Crimes and Violence Against Women (Dong, 2012). The historical origins of social policies directed toward the elder population are evidenced by the creation of Medicare, Medicaid, and the Older Americans Act (OAA), all becoming law in the 1960s (see Figure 3.1). The enactment of each of these federal laws has required public health administrators to be engaged in the three core public health functions as they provide services to the elder population.

Social Security Act

In developing the Social Security Act (SSA), which was signed into law in 1935, public health administrators were required to develop policies for successfully developing the program. This program is an example of implementing Public Health Law Model 4 and meeting the needs of elders through the concept of assurance. The SSA established the first federal assistance program for elders. The act provided resources to the states for assistance to elderly persons, along with benefits to retirees and the unemployed. Of special interest to EA are Titles XI, XVIII, XIX, and XX. Title XI created the requirement for reporting crimes in long-term care facilities to law enforcement. Title XVIII created the Medicaid provision for nursing facilities to recruit skilled and trained nursing personnel. Under Title XIX, nursing homes and community care facilities were directed to care for functionally disabled elderly individuals, and Title XX created block grants for social services and elder justice (SSA, n.d.). Under the

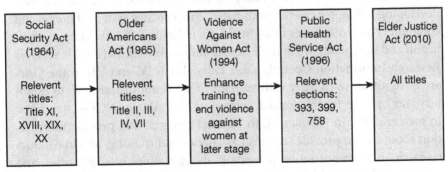

Figure 3.1 Development of legal policies associated with elder abuse.

SSA, public health administrators have a duty to provide safe facilities for elders under the act's provisions.

Adult Protective Services

In keeping with Public Health Law Model 5, APS was created by Title XX of the SSA, authorizing protective services for adults aged 18 years and older at all income levels who were experiencing abuse, neglect, or exploitation (Teaster, Wangmo, & Anetzberger, 2010). To assist victims of elder mistreatment, APS relies on a network of well-coordinated interdisciplinary social and health services. Because APS was developed during a period when insufficient data were available concerning elder mistreatment, the Title XX legislation appears to be pragmatic in nature (National Adult Protective Services Association, n.d.). The organization of APS varies by state, sometimes being under the oversight of county and human services agencies, designated as Departments of Health and Human Services, Social Services, or Family Services. In these instances, public health administrators are responsible for providing assurance that the provisions of the law are carried out and that elders are protected.

Older Americans Act

Demonstrating the use of Public Health Law Models 2 and 5, the OAA was enacted in 1965. This law, which focuses on the field of aging, authorizes state grants for research, community planning programs, and training projects. Many of these grants are within the purview of public health organizations at the state and local levels. Public health administrators are engaged in assessment of the needs of elders and developing the policies and regulations that are required to enable elders to obtain the required services. The OAA created the ACL, earlier named the AoA. The ACL was charged with developing a comprehensive, coordinated, cost-effective system of home- and community-based services to assist elderly individuals in maintaining their health and independence in their homes and communities (Health Services Research Information Central, n.d.). Titles II, III, IV, and VII of the OAA are of significance to elder mistreatment. Title II authorizes ACL to establish and operate the National Center on Elder Abuse (NCEA; described in greater detail in Chapter 7), to conduct research and provide information about EA, to provide technical assistance and training, and to conduct research and demonstration projects to develop objectives, priorities, and long-term plans for elder justice activities. Title III requires states that desire services from the NCEA to develop a plan to assure that the AoA programs will align with relevant state law and existing state APS-related activities. Through Title IV, ACL distributes grant funding for projects related to EA (OAA 2006, n.d.). The OAA is the major vehicle for the delivery of programs to the elderly population.

Long-Term Care Ombudsmen

One of the stipulations of the OAA is that every state is required to have an Ombudsman Program that addresses complaints and advocates for improvements in the long-term care system (National Long-Term Care Ombudsman Resource Center, n.d.). The AoA coordinates the ombuds network, and most states' ombuds programs are housed in their respective state units on aging. Typically, long-term care ombuds advocate for elderly individuals who are residents of nursing homes and assisted living facilities. They provide information for finding appropriate facilities and obtaining quality care. In 2011, the Long-Term Care Ombudsman Program investigated more than 200,463 complaints on behalf of 131,078 individuals and provided information about long-term care for an additional 288,698 people nationally (National Long-Term Care Ombudsman Resource Center, n.d.). This approach to elder care uses Public Health Law Model 6 because tort claims may be filed by state ombuds agencies to provide for the protection of elders.

The Eldercare Locator was developed under the OAA as a national service for identifying local and state Area Agencies on Aging. This program provides public and private assistance to elders at the local level, often through local public health departments. Funded through Title II of the OAA, the NCEA is a national resource center dedicated to the prevention of elder mistreatment. The NCEA provides public health program and policy development assistance, training and technical assistance, professional development opportunities, and a training library for personnel dealing with APS and elder mistreatment (National Center on Elder Abuse, n.d.). Because Public Health Law Model 2 encompasses altering the informational environment, the OAA provides highly useful information for the care of elders.

Elder Justice Act

The Elder Justice Act (EJA) was passed as Title VI, Section H of the Patient Protection and Affordable Care Act in 2010. The EJA authorizes a federal response to EA through training, services, demonstration programs, and the establishment of forensic centers to support collaborative efforts by legal, medical, social services, and law enforcement agencies directed toward the prevention and prosecution of crimes against the elderly. Although program funding relies on funds that have not yet been appropriated, the legislation used Public Health Law Model 1 to authorize the expenditure of necessary federal funds to implement the law and provide benefits to elders nationwide.

Part I of EJA requires the formation of an Elder Justice Coordinating Council, comprising federal government representatives charged with the responsibility of administering programs for the promotion of elder justice. The Council is tasked with providing recommendations to the Secretary of the DHHS on issues of abuse, neglect, and exploitation of the elderly. Part II of the EJA focuses on the authorization of programs aimed at enhancing long-term care, with a significant emphasis on state and local APS initiatives. Funding for programs enhancing the capacity of ombuds to report and resolve complaints of abuse, neglect, and exploitation of older adults were authorized, along with program development for recruiting and retaining long-term care staff; improving long-term care management practices; and assisting long-term care facilities in acquisition and implementation of electronic health record (EHR) technology.

PUBLIC HEALTH FRAMEWORK TO ADDRESS ELDER ABUSE

The administration of public health is concerned with providing the leadership and management at the population level to assist in the control and containment of known or developing population risks. Any issue that has a significant impact on a large portion of the American population, such as elders, is a public health issue. Public health administrators at the national, state, and local levels have the specific tasks under public health law to assess the health and well-being of elders and, based on their assessment, to develop the policies that are required to alleviate the issues identified. Such policies may result in either the development of new laws, ordinances, or regulations, or the deregulation (Public Health Law Model 7) of existing but inadequate rules and procedures, either in statutes or regulations.

Although there is no formula or framework used to apply a public health interprofessional approach to address EA, on the basis of the core functions of public health and the essential public health services discussed earlier, a crude framework such as PDSP may be applied.

POLICY BOX

As noted in the illustrative case study later in this chapter, it is not always easy to develop policy or legislation to provide support to the elder population, and doing so at the local level may be just as difficult. The Commonwealth of Kentucky has enacted legislation that provides the basis on which local public health policies can be developed. KRS (Kentucky Revised Statutes) 209.030 (11) states, "The cabinet (Cabinet of Health and Family Services) shall consult with local agencies and advocacy groups, including but not limited to long-term care ombudsmen, law enforcement agencies, bankers, attorneys, providers of nonemergency transportation services, and charitable and faith-based organizations, to encourage the sharing of information, provision of training, and promotion of awareness of adult abuse, neglect, and exploitation, crimes against the elderly, and adult protective services."[1] Clearly, the statute anticipates that the Cabinet will engage a broad coalition of providers, advocates, and governmental organizations in these core activities. However, each local jurisdiction also has the responsibility for bringing the appropriate broad coalition of individuals and groups together to carry out the legislative mandate. Often, the first issue to be resolved locally requires a determination of who or what organization will convene the policy group, including deciding the composition of group itself. Developing local policies and procedures to share information, provide training, and promote awareness of EA should be the end result of the group's effort.

---

[1] http://www.lrc.ky.gov/statutes/statute.aspx?id=8182

Identify prevalence: This step is related to the assessment core function, in which public health administrators regularly and systematically collect, assemble, and analyze community-based data concerning elder health and well-being. In this step, the questions investigated pertain to the trend of the specific condition in the community. Questions may include trends in the prevalence of the condition. A distribution analysis may be performed to determine the proportion of persons in the elder population who are affected by the situation, and whether that proportion is increasing or decreasing.

Diagnose the condition: This step addresses the third essential public health service, in which public health agencies are tasked with investigating and identifying community health hazards. The individual elements that may be investigated include the impact of a condition on the elder's ability to access services and facilities, the ability to perform normal social roles, and the pain and discomfort resulting from the condition.

Examine societal impact: This function inspects the effect of a condition across the elder community, which relates to the policy development core function. Within this function, public health administrators participate in the development of comprehensive public health policies that assess the economic impact of the condition. Examples include the effect of a condition on the economic performance of elders and the cost of care to those affected by the condition.

Assure preventability: This step is a public health approach in which the potential for prevention and treatment of a condition affecting elders is of interest. Here, the natural history of a condition such as financial abuse is taken into consideration, thereby enabling the detection of the condition at an early stage. Efforts are made to identify or develop interventions that resolve the condition. This step relates to the core public health function of assurance, in which public health administrators assure their communities that services required to contain the progress of the condition are available.

DISCUSSION BOX

The local public health agency of Nicholasville in central Kansas has an aging program through which agency personnel systematically collect, assemble, and analyze well-being data of local elders. Dorothy, a retired corporate executive assistant in her late 70s, is in the databases. She is quite alert and socially engaged, even though she is nearly 80 years of age. Since the death of her husband, Dorothy's designated caregiver has been her son. The aging program offered Dorothy and her son the option to hire nursing care from the local health agency, an offer they accepted. Dorothy also receives meals from the local "meals on wheels" program that maintains a log of her nutrition profile.

One day, Dorothy suffers a bad fall at home. Because the nurse comes only on alternate days, no one is at her home and her son has already left for work. She lies in pain inside her home, not knowing when help can be expected. It happens that the incident occurs on the day the home health inspector is scheduled for a visit. The inspector knocks at the door, but hears no response. Just as he is about to leave,

---

(continued)

DISCUSSION BOX *(continued)*

a "meals on wheels" volunteer arrives to deliver Dorothy's meal. When the home health inspector informs him that no one is at home, the meal provider informs the inspector that this could not be possible because he was scheduled to deliver the food. As per protocol, the food provider informs the program manager, who in turn checks in with the son. After confirming with the son that Dorothy was at home, the program manager informs the local police, who open the door and find Dorothy lying unresponsive on the floor. They immediately call 911 and emergency services take charge of the situation.

When Dorothy is taken to the emergency room, the hospital is able to access a log of her health status because it was maintained at the local public health agency by the nursing program. The home health inspector recommends installation of emergency systems that connect Dorothy with the local assistance authorities. Through the collective actions of several public health agencies that address the health needs of the elder population, the plan for caring for Dorothy was expedited.

The PDSP framework supports a public health administration approach to contain EA. In the first step, the prevalence of abuse in the elderly population is identified. For example, the national EA incidence report estimates that female elders are more likely than male elders to be mistreated and suggests that the older the individual, the higher the likelihood of mistreatment (National Center on Elder Abuse & American Public Human Services Association, 1998). Unfortunately, even given the recent attention to EA, prevalence and incidence rates are not as well known, especially because only one in 14 cases of EA comes to the attention of the authorities (U.S. National Research Council Panel to Review Risk and Prevalence of Elder Abuse and Neglect, Bonnie, & Wallace, 2003).

In the second step, the reason why EA is a significant problem is determined. According to *Profile of Older Americans*, the population aged 65 years and older is projected to more than double from 43 million people in 2012 to 92 million people in 2060. By 2040, there will be approximately 80 million older persons, more than twice the number in 2000. People aged 65 years and older represented 13.7% of the U.S. population in 2012, but are expected to account for 21% of the population by 2040. The population aged 85 years and older is projected to triple from 6 million in 2012 to 14 million in 2040 (AoA, 2013). This increase in the elder population, coupled with the high potential that almost all older adults will have at least one informal care provider (AoA, 2013), will result in a highly vulnerable population, especially given that earlier studies have suggested that the more elderly individuals in the population, the more likely they are to be mistreated (National Center on Elder Abuse & American Public Human Services Association, 1998).

In the third step, the societal impact of EA is examined. The cost of late-life dependency is projected to increase, as an older population cohort with fewer economic resources is expected to have substantial life care needs (AoA, 2013).

In the final step, preventability of the condition is considered. Studies have identified that policies to improve long-term services and reduce unmet support needs could benefit both older adults and those who care for them (Freedman & Spillman, 2014). Consequently, policy development engaged in by public health administrators can significantly control the incidence of EA if local, state, and federal governments enable elders to maintain their health in a healthy environment by committing resources to develop workforce capacity and build infrastructure dedicated to elder care.

Case Study: Enacting Adult Protective Services in Kentucky

In the 2004 legislative session of the Commonwealth of Kentucky General Assembly, a majority party member of the House of Representatives submitted a bill to establish APS in the Commonwealth of Kentucky. In December 2003, a new gubernatorial administration had been sworn in, and a governmental reorganization was under way in which the Cabinet for Children and Family Services and the Cabinet for Health Services were being combined into a single Cabinet for Health and Family Services (CHFS). It soon became apparent that the two former cabinets had not agreed on the substance of the bill. As a consequence, the newly appointed Cabinet Secretary refused to endorse the bill, creating a major disagreement with a powerful state representative. With the governorship and state Senate in the control of one political party and the state House of Representatives controlled by another party, it quickly became apparent that the bill was dead for the 2004 legislation session.

The Cabinet Secretary, recognizing the importance of enacting legislation protecting elders, offered to establish a bipartisan task

(continued)

Case Study: Enacting Adult Protective Services in Kentucky *(continued)*

force composed of cabinet officials, senators, and representatives of both political parties and organized groups advocating for elders and APS. As a result of the determined efforts and strong support of all members of the task force, a strong APS bill (HB 298, an Act Pertaining to the Protection of Adults) was introduced on February 2, 2005, in the Kentucky House of Representatives by the majority party. With the strong support of the Cabinet Secretary working with and through the Kentucky Senate, the bill was enacted by unanimous votes in both legislative chambers and signed into law by the governor on March 18, 2005.

Key provisions of the bill required the CHFS to "(a) specify cabinet actions upon receipt of a report to include notice to law enforcement within 24 hours and immediate notice when an emergency circumstance or a potential crime occurs; (b) require the cabinet to establish standardized procedures for notifying other authorized agencies; (c) if practical, require the cabinet to coordinate investigations with other agencies and to support specialized multidisciplinary teams with professionals who have investigative authority; (d) specify that cabinet representatives will be allowed access to financial records in an active investigation; (e) require the cabinet to consult with agencies and advocacy programs to encourage information sharing, training, and awareness of adult abuse, neglect, and exploitation; (f) require each agency that receives notice of a report from the cabinet to submit an annual report of actions taken and the current status of investigations; (g) require the cabinet to summarize all reports from other agencies into a report to the Governor and Legislature."[2]

In addition to enacting an important piece of legislation impacting the lives of elders throughout the Commonwealth of Kentucky, the teamwork developed through this process resulted in a strong bipartisan coalition dedicated to protecting elders.

---

[2] Kentucky Legislature. (2005). HB298: An Act Relating to the Protection of Adults. Retrieved from http://www.lrc.ky.gov/lrcsearch

SUMMARY

The magnitude of EA is quite significant, and EA remains an underappreciated public health issue despite the increasing trend in EA reporting and the institution of federal policies. Because of its complex nature, EA requires an interdisciplinary approach on the part of public health. Public health agencies, by their very nature and organizational structure, are well positioned to help address the issue of EA through the core functions of assessment, policy development, and assurance and the 10 essential services of public health. Public health administration is at the heart of the public health system, allowing highly skilled individuals the opportunity to assess the issues facing the health and well-being of elders, develop and implement policies to effectively deal with the issues discovered, and assure that elders are truly protected as they age.

The historical development of public health legal policies demonstrates that continued efforts need to be directed at expediting policy development. One way to facilitate policy development is through empirical, evidence-based policy development research. The PDSP framework can be applied by public health administrators to the issue of EA to highlight the population-level effect of the issue and to draw out the socioeconomic impact of EA on local communities and the nation as a whole. As more agencies recognize the need for collecting and using data on EA, more rigorous quantitative and qualitative studies will be conducted in the American context. Robust data sources, in combination with governmental support to encourage studies to contain and control the incidence of EA and an interdisciplinary approach involving public health administration, is a highly effective means of addressing the issue of EA.

Thought-Provoking Questions

1. Does the mission of your local public health department include protection of elders from abuse? If not, which steps can you take to change its mission?

2. The three core functions of public health, assessment, policy development, and assurance provide a logical framework for engaging public health on issues of EA. How would you apply this framework to a financial issue involving elders?

3. After reviewing the 10 essential public health services, how would you use them as a framework for engaging the public concerning the issue of EA in your community? For this purpose, which services are the most important?

4. In your work context, how can you use the PDSP framework to develop public health policy for EA? Which data are required in doing so?

5. Which individuals or groups should you include in your task group to draft new public health policies or legislation to provide support for your elder population? In your local community, are new public health policies required to identify, prevent, or treat EA? Is your local public health department engaged in such efforts?

REFERENCES

Acierno, R., Hernandez, M. A., Amstadter, A. B., Resnick, H. S., Steve, K., Muzzy, W., & Kilpatrick, D. G. (2010). Prevalence and correlates of emotional, physical, sexual, and financial abuse and potential neglect in the United States: The National Elder Mistreatment Study. *American Journal of Public Health, 100*(2), 292–297. doi:10.2105/AJPH.2009.163089

Administration on Aging. (2013). A profile of older Americans: 2013. Retrieved from   https://www.acl.gov/sites/default/files/Aging%20and%20Disability%20 in%20America/2013_Profile.pdf

Bonnie, R. J., & Wallace, R. B. (2003). *Elder mistreatment: Abuse, neglect, and exploitation in an aging America.* Washington, DC: National Academies Press. Retrievedfromhttp://search.ebscohost.com/login.aspx?direct=true&scope=site& db=nlebk&db=nlabk&AN=86940

Boyle, P. A., Barnes, L. L., Buchman, A. S., & Bennett, D. A. (2009). Purpose in life is associated with mortality among community-dwelling older persons. *Psychosomatic Medicine, 71*(5), 574–579. doi:10.1097/ PSY.0b013e3181a5a7c0

Bunker, J. P., Frazier, H. S., & Mosteller, F. (1994). Improving health: Measuring effects of medical care. *Milbank Quarterly, 72*(2), 225. doi:10.2307/3350295

CDC Foundation. (n.d.). What is public health? Retrieved from http://www .cdcfoundation.org/content/what-public-health

CDC Foundation. (n.d.). What is public health? Retrieved from https://www .cdcfoundation.org/blog-entry/value-public-health-protection-healthy -nation-2030

Centers for Disease Control and Prevention. (n.d.). Elder Abuse: Definitions. Retrieved from https://www.cdc.gov/violenceprevention/elderabuse/definitions.html

Centers for Disease Control and Prevention (CDC). (2007). *National public health performance standards program.* Washington, DC: Author. Retrieved from http://www.cdc.gov/NPHPSP/PDF/UserGuide.pdf

Committee on Assuring the Health of the Public in the 21st Century. (2002). *The future of the public's health in the 21st Century.* Washington, DC: Institute of Medicine. Retrieved from http://www.iom.edu/Reports/2002/The-Future-of -the-Publics-Health-in-the-21st-Century.aspx

DeBuono, B. A., & Tilson, H. E. (2003). *Advancing healthy populations: The Pfizer guide to careers in public health.* New York, NY: Pfizer Global Pharmaceuticals.

Dong, X. (2012). Advancing the field of elder abuse: Future directions and policy implications. *Journal of the American Geriatrics Society, 60*(11), 2151–2156. doi:10.1111/j.1532-5415.2012.04211.x

Ferris State University. (n.d.). Understanding Public Health and Health Care System Administration. Retrieved March 18, 2018, from https://ferris.edu/HTMLS/ colleges/alliedhe/PublicHealth/pdfs-docs/Understanding_Public_Health_ and_HCSA.pdf

Freedman, V. A., & Spillman, B. C. (2014). Disability and care needs among older Americans. *Milbank Quarterly, 92*(3), 509–541. doi:10.1111/1468-0009 .12076

Fulmer, T. T., & O'Malley, T. A. (1987). *Inadequate care of the elderly: A health care perspective on abuse and neglect.* New York, NY: Springer Publishing.

Goodman, R. A., Hoffman, R. E., Lopez, W., Matthews, G. W., Rothstein, M., & Foster, K. (Eds.). (2007). *Law in public health practice.* New York, NY: Oxford University Press. Retrieved from http://www.oxfordscholarship.com/view/10.1093/ acprof:oso/9780195301489.001.0001/acprof-9780195301489

Gostin, L. O., & Wiley, L. F. (2007). *Public health law: Power, duty, restraint* (2nd ed.). New York, NY: University of California Press and Milbank Memorial Fund. Retrieved from http://www.ucpress.edu/book.php?isbn=9780520253766

Hall, J. E., Karch, D. L., & Crosby, A. E. (2016). *Elder abuse surveillance: Uniform definitions and recommended core data elements for use in elder abuse surveillance, version 1.0.* Atlanta, GA: National Center for Injury Prevention and Control, Centers for Disease Control and Prevention.

Halverson, P. K., Miller, C. A., Kaluzny, A. D., Fried, B. J., Schenck, S. E., & Richards, T. B. (1996). Performing public health functions: The perceived contribution of public health and other community agencies. *Journal of Health and Human Services Administration, 18*(3), 288–303.

Health Services Research Information Central. (n.d.). Key organizations. Retrieved from http://www.nlm.nih.gov/hsrinfo/keyorganizations.html

Institute of Medicine (IOM). (n.d.). *Elder abuse and its prevention: A workshop.* Washington, DC. Retrieved from http://www.iom.edu/Activities/Global/

ViolenceForum/2013-APR-17/Day%201/Welcome%20and%20Early%20 Presentations/1-Welcome-Video.aspx

Institute of Medicine & Committee for the Study of the Future of Public Health. (1988). *The future of public health*. Washington, DC: National Academies Press- Retrieved from https://www.nap.edu/read/1091/chapter/1.

Lee, L. M. (2012). Public health ethics theory: Review and path to convergence. *Journal of Law, Medicine & Ethics, 40*(1), 85–98. doi:10.1111/ j.1748-720X.2012.00648.x

Lifespan of Greater Rochester, Weill Cornell Medical Center of Cornell University, & New York City Department for the Aging. (2011). *Under the radar: New York State Elder Abuse Prevalence Study*. New York, NY: Author. Retrieved from http://www.lifespan-roch.org/documents/undertheradar051211.pdf

Mather, M., Jacobsen, L. A., & Pollard, K. M. (2015). Ageing in the United States. *Population Bulletin,* 70(2), 2–18. Retrieved from https://www.prb.org/ wp-content/uploads/2016/01/aging-us-population-bulletin-1.pdf

Mays, G., Miller, C., & Halverson, P. (2000). *Local public health practice: Trends and models*. Washington, DC: American Public Health Association.

Modeste, N., & Tamayose, T. (2004). *Dictionary of public health promotion and education: Terms and concepts* (2nd ed.). San Francisco, CA: Jossey-Bass.

National Adult Protective Services Association. (n.d.). Elder Justice Act imple- mentation. Retrieved from http://www.napsa-now.org/policy-advocacy/eja -implementation/

National Center on Elder Abuse (NCEA). (n.d.). Who we are: NCEA history. Retrieved from https://ncea.acl.gov/whoweare/history.html

National Center on Elder Abuse & American Public Human Services Association. (1998). *The National Elder Abuse Incidence Study: Final report*. National Cen- ter on Elder Abuse. Retrieved from https://www.acl.gov/sites/default/files/ programs/2016-09/ABuseReport_Full.pdf

National Long-Term Care Ombudsman Resource Center. (n.d.). About ombuds- men. Retrieved from http://ltcombudsman.org/about/about-ombudsman

National Research Council (U.S.), Panel to Review Risk and Prevalence of Elder Abuse and Neglect, Bonnie RJ, Wallace RB. *Elder Mistreatment Abuse, Neglect, and Exploitation in an Aging America*. Washington, DC: National Academies Press; 2003. http://search.ebscohost.com/login.aspx?direct=true&scope=site& db=nlebk&db=nlabk&AN=86940. Accessed October 11, 2014.

Older Americans Act 2006. Retrieved from https://www.govtrack.us/congress/ bills/109/hr6197/text

Patient Protection and Affordable Care Act, Public Law, (111–148). (2010). Retrieved from http://legcounsel.house.gov/Comps/Patient%20Protection%20 And%20Affordable%20Care%20Act.pdf

Paul K, H. (2002). Embracing the strength of the public health system: why strong government public health agencies are vitally necessary but insufficient. *Journal of Public Health Management Practice, 8*(1), 98–100.

Quinn, M. J., & Tomita, S. K. (1997). *Elder abuse and neglect: Causes, diagnosis, and intervention strategies.* New York, NY: Springer.

Rowe, J. W., & Kahn, R. L. (1999). *Successful aging.* New York, NY: Dell.

Schmutzler, D. J., & Holsinger, J. W. (2011). New professionalism. In D. Bhugra & A. Malik (Eds.), *Professionalism in mental healthcare: Experts, expertise, and expectations.* Cambridge, UK: Cambridge University Press.

Shakespeare, W. (2004). *As you like it.* New York, NY: Simon & Schuster.

Singh, M. P. (2005). *Quote unquote: A handbook of quotations.* New Delhi, India: Lotus Press.

Social Security Act. (n.d.). Compilation of the Social Security Laws. Retrieved from http://www.ssa.gov/OP_Home/ssact/title09/0900.htm

Steinmetz, S. K. (1988). Elder abuse by family caregivers: Processes and intervention strategies. *Contemporary Family Therapy, 10*(4), 256–271. doi:10.1007/BF00891617

Taylor, R. M. (2013). Elder abuse and its prevention: Workshop summary. Retrieved from http://www.ncbi.nlm.nih.gov/books/NBK189833/pdf/TOC.pdf

Teaster, P. B., Dugar, T. A., Mendiondo, M. S., Abner, E. L., Cecil, K. A., & Otto, J. M. (2004). *The 2004 survey of state Adult Protective Services: Abuse of adults 60 years of age and older.* Washington, DC: National Center on Elder Abuse. Retrieved from http://www.ncea.aoa.gov/Resources/Publication/docs/APS_2004NCEA Survey.pdf

Teaster, P. B., Wangmo, T., & Anetzberger, G. J. (2010). A glass half full: The dubious history of elder abuse policy. *Journal of Elder Abuse & Neglect, 22*(1–2), 6–15. doi:10.1080/08946560903436130

U.S. Department of Health and Human Services. (n.d.). Home page. Retrieved from http://www.hhs.gov

U.S. National Research Council Panel to Review Risk and Prevalence of Elder Abuse and Neglect, Bonnie, R. J., & Wallace, R. B. (2003). *Elder Mistreatment Abuse, Neglect, and Exploitation in an Aging America.* Washington, DC: National Academies Press. Retrieved from https://www.ncbi.nlm.nih.gov/books/NBK98802/pdf/Bookshelf_NBK98802.pdf

World Health Organization (WHO). (2002). *World report on violence and health.* Geneva, Switzerland: Author.

World Health Organization (WHO). (n.d.). World report on knowledge for better health. Retrieved from http://www.who.int/rpc/meetings/wr2004/en/index8.html

4

INTIMATE PARTNER VIOLENCE AFFECTING OLDER ADULTS: PUBLIC HEALTH IMPLICATIONS

Holly Ramsey-Klawsnik

Intimate partner violence (IPV) is a multidimensional problem that requires interdisciplinary interventions and unfortunately has been overlooked for the older adult population. IPV usually escalates in severity and consequences during adults' later years, so it is critical that it is not mistakenly attributed to caregiver stress. Related topics such as polyvictimization have sometimes gone unrecognized by professionals who work with elderly victims—a problem that can result in delays or omissions in receiving assistance and needed support. All healthcare providers who provide services to older adults, including health and mental healthcare professionals and para-professionals and staff of aging services agencies and residential care facilities, need to be trained about this issue. Collaboration among involved service providers is essential.

IPV is a multifaceted and complex problem at the intersection of elder abuse (EA; e.g., commonly concerning the neglect and abuse of fragile and dependent elders) and domestic violence (e.g., commonly concerning younger victims and families/relationships). There is a critical need for practitioners in both fields to better understand and address this problem.

Chapter Objectives

By the end of this chapter, readers will be able to

1. Understand the multidimensionality of IPV related to older adults.

2. Describe why and how the IPV of older adults is a public health issue.

3. Explore how public health professionals can identify and respond to the IPV of older adults.

4. Examine cases of IPV involving older adults to understand case dynamics as well as how to maximize outcomes of prevention and intervention.

5. Understand how public health professionals can work with other professionals who intervene in cases involving IPV and older adults.

"Intimate partner violence includes physical violence, sexual violence, stalking and psychological aggression (including coercive tactics) by a current or former intimate partner" (Breiding, Basile, Smith, Black, & Mahendra, 2015). Although IPV reports decrease as the age of victims increases (Rennison, 2001), evidence reveals that IPV affects a substantial number of older adults. For example, Adult Protective Services (APS) data from 10 states revealed that 11% of the substantiated reports of abuse of persons aged 60 and older with a known perpetrator involved a spouse or intimate partner (Teaster et al., 2006).

As pointed out by Desmarais and Reeves (2007), incidents of IPV affecting older victims are often obscured by their inclusion under the broad definition of EA. IPV cases targeting older victims certainly constitute EA; however, failing to also identify them as cases of domestic abuse or IPV has contributed to a societal-wide tendency to overlook IPV affecting older adults. As a result, cases go unrecognized and, in turn, there is a dearth of IPV prevention and intervention strategies and initiatives aimed at older victims. This chapter presents and analyzes situations that were reported as alleged EA to APS programs in various states. All were confirmed as EA following investigations.[1] The goals are (a) to illustrate abuse and clinical dynamics of

---

[1] These actual cases came to the author's attention in her role as a clinical consultant for the APS programs that handled them. All identifying data have been removed or altered to protect the confidentiality and safety of those involved.

cases that constitute both EA and IPV, and (b) to illuminate the public health implications of EA cases that involve IPV affecting older adults.

ILLUSTRATIVE CASES

Long-Term IPV

The following case illustrates a common pattern of IPV in later years often referred to as "domestic violence grown old." In this pattern, victimization begins early in an intimate relationship and continues throughout the life course of the partners. In the following case, an adult son sought help for his mother, whom he had witnessed his father assault throughout his childhood.

> Sixty-year-old Mrs. V. has been married for forty-one years and is the mother of six children. . . Her son sought assistance for her due to marital rape. . . Mrs. V. acknowledged that throughout her marriage she had been repeatedly hit and forcibly sexually assaulted by her husband. There was also an extensive history of Mr. V. physically abusing the children. Although Mrs. V. had not been hit in many years, she was submissive to her husband and distraught about the continuing marital rape. Among the tactics used by Mr. V. to control his wife were prohibiting her from driving, working outside of the home, or managing money. (Ramsey-Klawsnik, 2003, p. 46)

Like Mrs. V., many older victims have sustained years of marital abuse that actually commenced decades before professional and public recognition of IPV, its profoundly harmful impact, and prevention and intervention strategies. When the assaults by her husband began 40 years earlier, Mrs. V. had no avenue for escape. Her religion, family, upbringing, values, and culture rendered her emotionally and realistically unable to seek separation or divorce from her abuser. She grew up in a social climate in which husbands were heads of households to be obeyed at all costs. She was not allowed to drive, and Mr. V. coercively controlled all money and other marital financial assets. The family resided in a rural area without public transportation that might facilitate escape. Furthermore, there was nowhere to go. Domestic violence shelters did not yet exist, and other entities that might have intervened did not exist or were not helpful.

Mrs. V. lacked family support because her parents and siblings had not immigrated to the United States. To further compound her lack of options, she had no formal education or means to independently support herself or her children. When the children were young and subjected to Mr. V.'s abuse, Child Protective Services were in their infancy. Mandatory child support had not yet evolved, so leaving her husband would have condemned Mrs. V. and her six children to a life of poverty. To save them and to survive, she endured more than 40 years of assaults, fear, and helplessness. When her son referred her to APS for assistance because of continuing marital abuse, Mrs. V. was suffering from major clinical depression, rarely spoke, and took no initiative in caring for herself or for her home. This evidence stood in sharp contrast to the "extremely hard-working mother" described by her son who, for years, spent every day washing, cooking, cleaning, attempting to keep her children safe, walking several miles daily carrying home groceries, and attempting to appease Mr. V. to avoid abuse to herself and the children. During investigative interviews, she confirmed enduring years of violent behavior by her husband directed at herself and her children. She was shocked to learn from involved abuse personnel that her husband's assaults constituted criminal behavior and that she had rights to protection under the law.

Public health implications:
Late-life IPV secondary prevention initiatives must aggressively educate older victims who were socialized prior to domestic violence legislation and services, as well as those who wish to protect them, about victim rights and available intervention strategies. These initiatives can also raise the awareness and understanding of domestic violence service personnel of the age and generational factors that may influence how IPV cases involving older adults can be effectively addressed.

Changes in Long-Term Domestic Violence

As illustrated by Mrs. V.'s case, domestic violence that has grown old may change during later years, with the amount of physical violence declining, but with other forms of coercive control being intensified to compensate and continue the coercive control. Despite these possible shifts and contrary to common assumptions, a key finding emerging from interviews with older victims is that domestic abuse often escalates in severity and consequences during later life. This is particularly likely when victims become ill or lose self-care abilities, as illustrated by the following scenario:

A Home Health Aide Agency reported to Adult Protective Services [about the] suspected abuse of 73-year-old Clara T. Mrs. T.

resides with her husband, Tom. She has had a stroke, experiences right-side paralysis, is nonambulatory, speaks with difficulty, and spends most of the time in a hospital bed set up in her dining room. Her home health aide reported the following: During a routine visit, Clara began to cry, stated that she did not feel well, and asked Tom to bring her a pain reliever. Tom gruffly responded by ordering Clara to "Shut up!" Clara's crying escalated. Tom picked up a pillow and approached his wife. He forcibly held the pillow over her face, and angrily stated that when he tells her to "shut up," that is what he expects her to do. (Ramsey-Klawsnik, 2000, p. 17)

The home health aide recognized this episode as EA, which required reporting it to her supervisor. During subsequent meetings between staff of the involved Visiting Nurse Association (VNA) and APS personnel who became involved, well-intended VNA staff expressed their belief that Mr. T. was a stressed and "overwhelmed caregiver." The nurses were of the opinion that the indicated intervention was to reduce his stress through referral to a caregivers' support group.

As pointed out by Brandl and Raymond (2012), "Studies show the causes of elder abuse to be wide-ranging—and not necessarily an outcome of caregiver stress. Seeing caregiver stress as a primary cause of abuse has unintended and detrimental consequences that affect the efforts to end this widespread problem" (p. 32). Applying the "caregiver stress" explanation to instances of late-life IPV is a form of ageism in which older adults as a group are viewed as dependent, difficult, and requiring inordinate amounts of care. This assumption also prevents examination of aspects of relationship dynamics and relationship history that must be accounted for when seeking to define actions most suited to protect older victims. "Notwithstanding the popular image of abuse arising from dependent victims and stressed caregivers, evidence is accumulating that neither caregiver stress levels nor victim levels of dependency may be core factors leading to elder abuse" (Wolf, 2000, p. 9). Often the abuse more typically mirrors the type of abuse suffered by younger battered women (Brandl et al., 2007).

The nurses' erroneous assumption that this was a case of caregiver stress was corrected during subsequent APS investigative interviews with Mrs. T. She stated that Tom had always been domineering and short-tempered and revealed a long history of physical, verbal, emotional, and sexual abuse. Since her stroke, she had been totally dependent on him for food, drink, medicine, bathing, dressing, toileting, and transferring from bed to chair, other than brief periods of home health service. Often Tom did not respond to her requests for assistance and became angry and rough on the occasions when he did. Furthermore, episodes of physical and sexual assault continued despite her debilitation. She was particularly distressed that she needed him to change her soiled undergarments because he frequently took sexual advantage of her at these times. To avoid forced sexual contact, she often remained for long periods of time in wet and soiled adult diapers. This caused painful and dangerous skin breakdown and infections that further complicated her fragile physical condition.

RESEARCH BOX

As described by Ramsey-Klawsnik et al. (2008), relatively little research has been undertaken on the problem of elder sexual abuse, and that which has been conducted has shed more light on the circumstances of the victims rather than the perpetrators. Ramsey-Klawsnik et al. examined a total of 429 cases of alleged sexual abuse of vulnerable adults living in care facilities investigated in five states (New Hampshire, Oregon, Tennessee, Texas, and Wisconsin) during a 6-month period (May 1, 2005 to October 31, 2005). In 103 cases (83%), there was one identified alleged sexual abuse perpetrator; two alleged perpetrators were identified in 8 cases (6.5%), totaling 119 alleged sexual perpetrators in the abuse reports investigated. The majority (73%) of the elder sexual abuse cases occurred in nursing homes, whereas 10% of the cases occurred in assisted living facilities. Other cases occurred in residential care facilities, community-based residential programs, rehabilitation centers, and state mental hospitals. Despite the fact that police were notified in the alleged cases, none of the 32 confirmed sexual perpetrators was arrested. In fact, only one of the alleged 119 elder sexual offenders faced arrest. An interesting finding is that women were confirmed as sexual perpetrators, which suggests that vulnerable elders receiving care in facilities must be protected from possible sexual offenders of both genders.

The authors conclude that to prevent sexual and other abuse of residents in care facilities, careful screening of potential employees and residents, checking criminal records, obtaining employment references, and skillful interviewing prior to accepting potential employees and residents are all critical measures. Diligent, ongoing supervision is also required for both employees and residents having access to

(continued)

vulnerable adults. Furthermore, individuals responsible for the safety of residents must be aware of the potential for visitors, including family members, to assault those receiving care—both in the facility as well as on outings away from the facility. All facility staff should be trained to recognize and appropriately respond to indicators of resident sexual abuse.

Public health implications:

1. *IPV often escalates in severity and consequences during later years, especially victims facing health problems and disabilities.*

2. *Secondary violence prevention efforts must inform healthcare and other professionals that abuse in later life is not primarily the result of caregiver stress. The caregiver stress model conveys that abuse inflicted by care providers is understandable and supports the perpetrator rather than the victim, which in turn is likely to exacerbate violence.*

3. *Late-life IPV adversely affects victims' health in ways beyond inflicted injuries. Victims who require care often experience dangerous neglect by their spouse perpetrators and forego care in an attempt to minimize the violence experienced.*

4. *Actions that victims take to avoid abuse may exacerbate or increase risks for other adverse health conditions.*

Older IPV Perpetrators with Disabilities

The previous case demonstrates the increased vulnerability to IPV of older adults who are seriously ill or disabled. A less visible reality is that some older IPV perpetrators have their own disabilities and care needs, as illustrated in the following situation:

Seventy-two-year-old Helen lived alone; her spouse, John, lived with a son and daughter-in-law due to his extensive care needs. Helen visited John once weekly, during which John demanded sexual contact. John would ask Helen to undress and then fondle her. Helen reported that she did not want this contact but feared that if she refused her husband would divorce her and cut her off financially. Helen was treated for depression by a psychiatrist. . . [who referred her to APS upon learning of this elder abuse].

During the [APS] investigation, Helen discussed feeling forced into unwanted sexual contact by her husband under the threat of being left totally without funds, as John had historically been the breadwinner and all financial assets were in his name. These threats had been an issue throughout the marriage. Demanding sexual relations from Helen had been a long-standing pattern. . . John admitted to demanding sex from his wife and felt that this was his right. Although he denied threatening to cut his wife off financially, he admitted to telling her she would have nothing without him. (Chihowski & Hughes, 2008, pp. 386–387)

John's admission of forcing his wife into sexual contact and sense of entitlement are consistent with research findings (Ramsey-Klawsnik, 2003) that many older men who sexually assaulted their wives admitted doing so and expressed that such behavior is acceptable.

Public health implications:

1. *Late-life IPV prevention strategies must aim to achieve societal-wide recognition that a marriage license (a) is not, in fact, a license to perpetrate abuse in any way, including forcing sexual contact, and (b) does not require any individual to endure spousal abuse or exploitation.*

2. *Targeted messages specifically for older adults are justified, given that certain segments of the older adult population may still hold ideas and views that might be conducive to abuse or that may thwart interventions.*

3. *Late-life IPV secondary prevention initiatives must include educating older perpetrators, who were socialized prior to domestic violence legislation, that harming spouse/partners is a criminal offense for which arrest of the perpetrator is mandatory.*

Clinical and research findings reveal that, similar to IPV involving younger people, most older victims of IPV are female and most older perpetrators are male. For example, Jasinski and Dietz (2003) found that older women were three times more likely to experience physical IPV than were men. However, and even less recognized, late-life IPV involving abuse of men by women does occur and is illustrated in the next case.

This case also provides an example of a victim who, despite poor health, serves as the perpetrator's care provider. Given the normal age-prevalent changes and increased health complications typically faced during the aging process, it is not unusual for both partners in an older couple to experience illnesses and compromised functioning. In many identified late-life IPV cases, victims provide care for their perpetrator despite their own health conditions and limitations. This case came forward for intervention when the victim discussed his plight with his healthcare provider:

> Eighty-year-old Mr. R. has been married to Silvia for over fifty years. He has a slight build and is treated for a prostate problem and clinical depression. He is mentally competent and intelligent. Seventy-nine-year-old Silvia is diagnosed with schizo-affective disorder and is described as anxious, irritable, and combative. She is 70 pounds overweight but claims to be anorexic. Silvia has experienced recurrent psychiatric hospitalizations, sees a therapist regularly, and is treated with psychotropic medication. Therapists for Mr. and Mrs. R. are concerned about Silva's treatment of her husband. Silvia orders Mr. R. to get up several times nightly to bring her food and demands that he stay awake while she eats. Silvia frequently becomes enraged with her husband and "pummels" him. Mr. R. is impotent, and Silvia regularly demands sexual intercourse. She becomes enraged when he does not perform, resulting in frequent physical assaults. Silvia has pulled her husband around the house by his penis and assaulted his penis and testicles on numerous occasions. She does not allow Mr. R. to leave the house without her. Mr. R. feels that Silvia's behavior is a result of her mental illness, and that it is his duty as her husband to take care of her. Mental health [and other services] are provided, however, Mrs. R.'s abusive behaviors continue. Mr. R. wants to remain in his marriage, but would like the abuse to end. (Ramsey-Klawsnik, 2003, pp. 48–49)

This case also provides insight regarding victims who feel compelled to remain with their perpetrators to provide needed care. Although afraid of Silvia and concerned for his personal safety, Mr. R.'s upbringing and values (and, in fact, his marriage vows) dictated loyalty toward and continued care provision of his ill spouse.

Mr. R. expressed a sentiment often heard from both male and female IPV victims—the desire to maintain the marriage but end the violence. This preference can be especially strong among older victims who have been married for decades. The emotional consequences of long-term IPV, including low self-esteem and resignation, create barriers to self-protection. Emotional, social, and financial attachments between spouses multiply over the years, making separation and/or divorce and "starting over" more daunting. The dissolution of a marriage at any age results in numerous practical problems. These challenges are significantly multiplied for older couples, especially when one or both partners experience care needs. As the illustrative cases reveal, older IPV victims with disabilities often rely upon their offenders to avoid nursing home or other facility placements. Conversely, many victims like Mr. R. feel a duty to provide care to ill and abusive spouses.

Public health implications:

1. *Late-life IPV involving male victims and female perpetrators must be recognized and addressed in prevention and intervention initiatives. The social norms that may prohibit disclosure or reporting of abuse by males must be recognized. It also must be borne in mind that male IPV victims may not have access to the same kinds or levels of resources that are typically available to female IPV victims, such as shelters.*

2. *Late-life IPV victims often provide care for their ill or disabled abusive spouses. Healthcare professionals and para-professionals routinely interact with and observe these couples and, therefore, are in an excellent position to identify and assist these victims.*

3. *Intervention strategies in cases of late-life IPV must address the health problems and care needs experienced by both victims and perpetrators.*

4. *Interventionists must recognize and appreciate that late-life IPV victims often face significant psychosocial barriers to leaving an abusive spouse.*

5. *Social messaging can serve as an important way to deter normative acceptance of these behaviors.*

Recent Onset of Domestic Violence in a New Relationship

Although the majority of identified late-life IPV cases involve "domestic violence grown old," there is another pattern of later-life IPV—namely, recent onset of IPV in a relatively new relationship. With increased life expectancy and socialization changes, older adults are increasingly engaged in dating, cohabitation, and remarriage. This pattern is demonstrated in the following case:

> Sixty-four-year-old Mrs. T. had been married for one year, following a month-long courtship. Several months into the marriage, Mrs. T. reported to her physician that her husband repeatedly hurt her during sex. The physician prescribed a vaginal cream. Mrs. T. further explained that her husband forced her to engage in sex acts that she did not like. The physician advised, "Just tell him no," and provided no further assistance. Several months later, Mrs. T. sought help from the director of her senior center. She confided that her husband demanded sex on a daily basis and frequently bruised her by grabbing and forcing sexual acts. The director filed a Protective Service report (as required by law), which was investigated. During forensic interviewing, Mrs. T. reported that her husband had an explosive temper and his sexual aggressiveness had escalated in recent months. She was particularly upset to be forced into oral sex, and was quite anxious and fearful because her husband was threatening to force anal sex. Evidence present included a bite mark on her right breast and various thumb and finger imprint bruises on her arms, thighs, and buttocks. Mrs. T. regretted the marriage and contemplated leaving her husband, but worried about the many problems this would create. (Ramsey-Klawsnik, 2003, p. 47)

In this case, investigative interviewing and attempts to assist the victim to safety plan were thwarted by the perpetrator's jealous and possessive behavior. He insisted upon accompanying Mrs. T. to all of her activities, including those at the senior center, and took extensive measures to minimize her opportunities to speak privately with others. He angrily accused her of having affairs

---

DISCUSSION BOX

Discuss how educating healthcare providers about late-life IPV has the potential to impact the outcomes of victims who choose to seek out help. Raising awareness about IPV in later life and teaching providers about the signs of IPV represent important steps to address it. Distinguishing caregiver stress from IPV and recognizing revictimization and polyvictimization are critical concepts to understand to prevent IPV and avoid victim-blaming.

if she found opportunity for a brief private conversation. This raised a host of complications for Mrs. T. and for the social services personnel attempting to assist her. The senior center director was extremely helpful in creating brief private opportunities for Mrs. T. to meet with those attempting to assist her.

This case illustrates harm inflicted when professionals miss or overlook abuse disclosures and fail victims needing assistance. The physician failed to comprehend and respond to Mrs. T.'s legitimate request for help with assaults that injured and terrified her. As a consequence, Mrs. T. felt unsupported, unassisted, and ashamed. She suffered continuing abuse before finding the courage, and opportunity, to seek help from her senior center director. The physician's instruction to Mrs. T. to "Just tell him [her abusive husband] no" revealed the healthcare provider's ignorance of both EA and IPV dynamics and consequences.

Public health implications:

1. *IPV training, although widely available, focuses on younger victims while overlooking older victim markers and primary and secondary prevention strategies. This conveys the erroneous message that IPV does not affect older people and leaves helping professionals unprepared to assist older victims or, worse, results in them providing dangerous or harmful interventions.*

2. *It must be recognized that attempts to assist an IPV victim may actually increase danger to that person. Extreme caution is required to carefully plan and problem-solve intervention attempts.*

3. *It is important to recognize and act in ways that acknowledge that more than individual acts by victims or by professionals are required to stop or prevent abuse. Relationship dynamics create circumstances in which singular persons may not have enough agency, resources, or wherewithal to change the circumstances faced. Response coordination must be carefully, comprehensively, and cohesively planned to reduce risks to all involved. Moreover, efforts to intervene must contain the right mixture of stakeholders to ensure that assistance can be provided both effectively and safely.*

Care Facility Placement for Older Victims with Disabilities

Intervention options for victims who have been forced to rely upon abusive spouse/partners to meet complex care needs are indeed limited. One alternative is placement in a nursing home or other long-term care facility to escape IPV. The victim described in the following case eventually requested this option.

> A 78-year-old woman with Parkinson's disease resided at home with her husband, who was her primary care provider. A report to APS resulted in the determination that the husband was emotionally abusive and neglectful of his wife. Service providers became involved, including a physical therapist to provide home-based therapy to the wife. Upon one visit, the husband literally dragged his wife out of the bedroom, kicking her feet to force her to move faster. He berated her for being slow and clumsy. The therapist was shocked and deeply concerned upon witnessing this. She instantly realized that she would need to report this to the involved APS caseworker, but did not know how to immediately respond. Horrified, she watched, fearing that attempting to intervene or correct the husband would lead to escalated abuse when she left the premises. (Ramsey-Klawsnik, 2007, pp. 19–20)

Unfortunately, as she left the home, the physical therapist commented, "I can see that your wife is hard to take care of" in the presence of both the husband and wife. This statement demoralized the wife, who felt blamed for her own abuse, unsupported, and revictimized by the therapist. The abusive husband interpreted this comment as the therapist's approval of his behavior. As a result, the secondary violence prevention efforts already under way were significantly derailed. A careful intervention plan was created in attempt to repair the damage. The physical therapist

> . . . was encouraged to discuss the incident with the wife upon her next visit, which was purposely scheduled during a time when the husband would be absent from the home. Suggestions provided included telling her client, "It looked like it was painful for you when your husband dragged you out of the bedroom and kicked your feet." When the therapist implemented the suggestion, the wife expressed strong emotion about her husband's behavior, stating that similar incidents occurred regularly. The therapist had also been coached to provide the messages, "I was so sorry to see you treated that way. I am sorry that I was unable to stop it or help you at that time. I feared that if I confronted him, he would become more abusive when I left. I want to let you know that I am very concerned for your safety. I have discussed the incident with your APS caseworker, and we want

to work with you to find solutions so that this will not continue." This conversation helped build a stronger therapeutic relationship and also facilitated discussion about the episode between the client and the APS worker. Ultimately, the case was resolved when the client stated, "I want to live in a place where they know how to take care of people." Placement in a quality care facility was arranged. (Ramsey-Klawsnik, 2007, p. 20)

Public health implications:

1. *Late-life IPV training, especially that designed for healthcare and related personnel, must include markers for case recognition, appropriate prevention and intervention strategies, and guidelines for responding to witnessed or disclosed IPV incidents in ways that best preserve and enhance victim safety.*

2. *Healthcare and related personnel must avoid reinforcing factors that may make disclosure of abuse or actions by victims to escape abuse less likely or unlikely.*

Unfortunately, Late-Life IPV May Continue Following Facility Placement

Older IPV victims who accept placement in residential care facilities find relief from depending on their abusers for basic necessities and daily care. Regrettably, case handling has revealed a distressing finding: IPV may continue even after an older victim enters a care facility. Stonehouse and Scahill (2012) provide an illustrative case.

The victim, 71-year-old "Mrs. Turner," had suffered several strokes that resulted in expressive aphasia (inability to speak) and paralysis requiring wheelchair use. She resided in a nursing facility, and her husband took her home for weekly visits. Facility staff repeatedly observed Mrs. Turner drag her feet in an attempt to block her husband from wheeling her chair out of the facility for visits home, although she did not display this behavior at other times. The distress that she repeatedly displayed in regard to going home with her husband resulted in the staff filing a report with state officials of suspected elder abuse. During careful interviewing by trained and experienced APS investigators, Mrs. Turner disclosed via writing, gesturing, pointing, and shaking her head "yes" or "no" that she did not want visits with her husband. She wrote and gestured to reveal that he physically and sexually assaulted her on visits home. She indicated that the violence was long-standing. Mrs. Turner's two adult daughters confirmed a long history of abuse by Mr. Turner dating back to their childhoods. Mrs. Turner very clearly communicated her wish for protection from her husband. Advocacy and protection measures were put in place through the collaborative efforts of the nursing home staff, APS personnel, the ombudsmen program, the local court that issued an order of protection and law enforcement personnel who enforced it, and the victims' daughters who provided emotional support and encouragement to their mother. Following a period of freedom from abuse, physical and speech therapy enabled Mrs. Turner to regain some ability to speak and bear weight. She was eventually discharged to the home of one of her daughters and filed for divorce.

Public health implications:

1. *In facilities caring for older adults who go out on visits home, staff training should be provided that calls attention to the possibility that abuse could occur during these visits. This training should also emphasize options or alternatives that could be implemented to reduce the likelihood that abuse might occur during such visits.*

2. *Health professionals and other care providers serving older adults in facilities, as well as in the community, must be trained to prevent, recognize, and respond to late-life IPV.*

3. *Investigative personnel such as APS workers and law enforcement officers need training in effective forensic interviewing methods for use with older suspected victims. When alleged victims experience disabilities, interviewers must adjust to the victim's limitations, abilities, and typical communication methods. Communication remedies, including nonverbal techniques, may be needed.*

4. *It is possible for older victims of EA and IPV, even those who have endured long-term abuse and experience disabilities, to achieve greater safety and improved mental and physical health.*

5. *The coordinated and collaborative efforts of multiple professionals and organizations are required to assist older IPV victims.*

6. *The value of family support for older IPV victims cannot be over-estimated.*

SUMMARY

Victimization of older adults by spouse/partners is a multifaceted and complex public health problem that constitutes both EA and IPV. The challenges faced by younger and older IPV victims are similar in many ways. These include societal, family, and, in some cases, religious pressures to fulfill marital vows, "until death do you part." The economic costs of separation and divorce and lack of housing and other resources also frequently impede IPV victims of all ages from seeking safety from violent partners.

There are also significant unique challenges confronted by older victims. The harmful physical consequences of IPV are multiplied for older victims because of normal age-prevalent physical changes, such as bones becoming more brittle and increased vulnerability to injury. The serious adverse health consequences of EA, which include physical harm, disability, increased hospitalization use, and increased mortality, have been well documented (see, for example, Dong & Simon, 2013). Research also confirms the increased adverse health consequences experienced by older IPV victims. For example, Zink, Fisher, Regan, and Pabst (2005) found that older female victims of IPV are more likely to report health problems than women of the same age who have not experienced IPV, and that they are physically injured in 45% of IPV events. It is important to note that adverse health conditions caused by IPV can involve permanent disability. This is vividly portrayed in the Office on Violence Against Women (2005) video, *In Their Own Words*, which depicts actual victim stories. One victim, Pat, a 50-year survivor of IPV that continued into her senior years, was struck by her husband in the knee with a police billy club. This assault left her with a lifelong disability requiring the use of a walker.

IPV typically inflicts tremendous psychological suffering on older victims, perhaps more than other types of EA (e.g., victimization by a paid care provider) because "Assault is more psychologically injurious when inflicted by someone expected to provide love, protection, and support" (Ramsey-Klawsnik, 2003, p. 57). IPV often worsens over time in nature and consequences, particularly when victims become ill or lose self-care abilities. Older adults who face physical challenges such as paralysis, or cognitive challenges such as dementia, may have a different subjective experience of an interpersonal assault and may experience more helplessness, shame, and self-blame than an older adult who does not (extrapolated from Burgess & Phillips, 2006).

Because of generational issues, older IPV victims often experience greater feelings of shame, blame, isolation, and hopelessness and powerlessness than younger victims socialized during or since the women's movement.

This social movement helped to bring about the availability of domestic violence shelters, restraining orders, mandatory domestic violence training for police, and mandatory perpetrator arrest, as well as increasing public and professional recognition of violence in the home by intimate partners. Older adults were often socialized in a climate that discriminated against women and afforded no legal protection from domestic violence, but instead blamed victims for their own abuses. There was little social support for women's right to protection from domestic violence and no protection from marital rape under the law. Furthermore, individuals who have experienced decades of domestic abuse typically suffer extensive psychosocial and physical damage, including extensive deterioration of self-esteem and disempowerment (Ramsey-Klawsnik, 2009, p. 5).

Services for IPV victims are largely unavailable to older adults. Accessing and using traditional intervention services, such as shelters, is particularly challenging for older adults with disabilities and/or cognitive loss. Effective and increased options for achieving safety are urgently needed for older IPV victims, including accessible, affordable, and safe housing.

Older IPV victims with disabilities often rely on their abusive spouses to avoid nursing home or other facility placements. Conversely, many older adults victimized by spouses with care needs feel unable to terminate the marriage because of a duty to care for their ill and abusive spouse.

Older IPV victims are, to a large extent, overlooked. Healthcare and other helping professionals are rarely trained to be alert and prepared for older IPV victims. For the most part, IPV outreach and public and professional education efforts do not target or even address older adults. IPV research, public awareness campaigns, and primary and secondary prevention efforts have generally not addressed older victims.

The illustrative cases presented demonstrate that late-life IPV typically involves "polyvictimization":

> Polyvictimization in later life occurs when a person aged 60 or older is harmed through multiple co-occurring or sequential types of elder abuse by one or more perpetrators, or when an older adult experiences one type of abuse perpetrated by multiple others with whom the older adult has a personal, professional, or care recipient relationship in which there is a societal expectation of trust. Perpetrators of polyvictimization in later life include individuals with special access to older adults, such as intimate partners; other family members; fiduciaries; and paid or unpaid care or service providers, resident(s), or service recipients in care settings. (Ramsey-Klawsnik & Heisler, 2014, p. 15)

A U.S. Department of Justice Office for Victims of Crime-funded project has found that polyvictimization in later life is a common, complex, multidimensional problem that must be addressed comprehensively. The project authors recommend that responses and interventions be victim-centered and trauma-informed (Ramsey-Klawsnik & Miller, 2017).

The illustrative cases presented in this chapter reveal the large array of service providers who may potentially identify and respond to late-life IPV in helpful or harmful ways. These include health and mental health-care professionals and para-professionals and staff of aging services agencies and residential care facilities. Professionals specializing in services to older victims—in particular, APS and law enforcement personnel—need resources to adequately and safely respond in such cases. However, not just elder service providers but all providers who may interact with older adults require training in recognizing and responding to late-life IPV as a specific and highly dangerous form of EA. Very importantly, collaboration among involved service providers is essential (see Brandl et al., 2007, for guidance).

Informed and effective responses to IPV affecting younger adults can help to avert domestic violence "grown old." This, in turn, can reduce the long-term cumulative physical and psycho-social harm to adult victims and prevent trauma sustained by the children of affected families. However, as illustrated by the cases presented in this chapter, it is essential that public health initiatives aimed at preventing and reducing IPV incidents address victims and perpetrators throughout the age span, not just younger families, victims, and perpetrators as is the norm today.

IPV in later life is a complex and multifaceted problem that lies at the intersection of EA and domestic violence. Both fields have, in some ways, overlooked it, with EA-related efforts historically being focused primarily on abuse and neglect of fragile, dependent elders by overwhelmed care providers and domestic violence-related interventions focusing on much younger victims and families/relationships. There is a need for both fields to better understand the issue, develop resources and services, and learn from each other. At every juncture, public health deals with issues such as this, in which a multidimensional problem requires interdisciplinary interventions. If victimization of older adults by spouses/partners continues to be seen as something other than a public health problem, the "silver tsunami" of rapidly changing demographic patterns will suffer under its weight, and the human and financial costs of continuing the current pattern will increase dramatically.

POLICY BOX

The 1994 Violence Against Women Act (VAWA), with additions passed in 1996, outlined grant programs to prevent violence against women and established a national domestic violence hotline. In addition, new protections were given to victims of domestic abuse, such as confidentiality of a new address and changes to immigration laws that allow a battered spouse to apply for permanent residency. The act also addressed inter-state travel for the purposes of committing an act of domestic violence or violating an order of protection. A convicted abuser may not follow the victim into another state, nor may a con-victed abuser force a victim to move to another state. In earlier times, orders of protection issued in one jurisdiction were not always recognized in another jurisdiction; however, 47 states have now passed legislation that recognizes orders of protection issued in other jurisdictions. Three states—Alaska, Montana, and Pennsylvania—require that an out-of-state order be filed with an in-state jurisdiction before the order can be enforced. VAWA also allows victims of domestic abuse to sue for damages in civil court. Another goal of VAWA was to influence state legislators, particularly in regard to arrest policy for domes-tic situations. For example, to receive federal funding, states must adopt certain responses, such as implementing pro-arrest programs and policies in police departments, including manda-tory arrest programs and policies for protection order violations (Part U, SEC. 2101). This act has had a profound effect on state laws governing domestic abuse.[2]

---

[2] Federal Domestic Violence Legislation. (2013). The Violence Against Women Act, FindLaw. Retrieved from http://files.findlaw.com/pdf/family/family.findlaw.com_domestic-violence_federal-domestic-violence-legislation-the-violence-against-women.pdf

Thought-Provoking Questions

1. How can healthcare professionals be educated to recognize the signs of caregiver stress but avoid making the faulty assumption that caregiver stress is a major cause of EA? Which kinds of interventions could be designed to teach this topic to healthcare professionals and older adults?

2. Considering that older IPV victims face many barriers to leaving an abusive partner, which types of resources could be introduced to them? What are the safest and most effective ways to reach victims and also provide services to them?

3. Which cautions are required when attempting to reach victims to provide interventions? How can trusted family members be approached to assist in this process?

4. Who are the stakeholders in the topic of IPV? How can different stakeholders be engaged in a meaningful way to raise awareness and effectively prevent this form of abuse?

5. What are primary, secondary, and tertiary prevention strategies for IPV? Which of these strategies, if used in a wrong way, could have more harmful effects on the victims?

6. Which strategies could be used to prevent IPV in care facilities? Do you think using surveillance cameras to monitor the care of residents who have mental and physical disabilities conflicts with their privacy rights?

7. Which steps should care facility nurses and other staff take if they observe or otherwise suspect abuse of a resident?

8. Which types of health professionals could provide services to older adults who face multivictimization? How these professionals could work collaboratively to address such cases?

AUTHOR'S NOTE

For their careful reviews of and helpful suggestions to this chapter the author expresses appreciation to attorney Candace J. Heisler, expert trainer and consultant in elder abuse and IPV, and Dr. Joseph A. Klawsnik, clinical psychologist.

REFERENCES

Brandl, B., Dyer, C., Heisler, C., Otto, J., Stiegel, L., & Thomas, R. (2007). *Elder abuse detection and intervention: A collaborative approach.* New York, NY: Springer Publishing.

Brandl, B., & Raymond, J. (2012). Policy implications of recognizing that caregiver stress is not the primary cause of elder abuse. *Generations, 36*(3), 32–39.

Breiding, M. J., Basile, K. C., Smith, S. G., Black, M. C., & Mahendra, R. R. (2015). *Intimate partner violence surveillance: Uniform definitions and recommended data elements, version 2.0.* Atlanta, GA: National Center for Injury Prevention and Control, Centers for Disease Control and Prevention.

Burgess, A. W., & Phillips, S. L. (2006). Sexual abuse, trauma and dementia in the elderly: A retrospective study of 284 cases. *Victims & Offenders, 1*(2), 193–204. doi:10.1080/15564880600663935

Chihowski, K., & Hughes, S. (2008). Clinical issues in responding to alleged elder sexual abuse. *Journal of Elder Abuse & Neglect, 20*, 377–400. doi:10.1080/08946560802359383

Desmarais, S. L., & Reeves, K. A. (2007). Gray, black, and blue: The state of research and intervention for intimate partner abuse among elders. *Behavioral Sciences & the Law, 25*, 377–391. doi:10.1002/bsl.763

Dong, X., & Simon, M. A. (2013). Elder abuse as a risk factor for hospitalization in older persons. *JAMA Internal Medicine, 173*(10), 911–917. doi:10.1001/jamainternmed.2013.238

Jasinski, J. L., & Dietz, T. L. (2003). Domestic violence and stalking among older adults: An assessment of risk markers. *Journal of Elder Abuse & Neglect, 15*(1), 3–18. doi:10.1300/J084v15n01_02

Office for Victims of Crime. (2005). *In their own words: Domestic abuse in later life: Video and training guide.* (Publication No. 227928) Washington, DC: U.S. Department of Justice Office of Justice Programs and Terra Nova Films.

Ramsey-Klawsnik, H. (2000). Elder-abuse offenders: A typology. *Generations, 24*(2), 17–22.

Ramsey-Klawsnik, H. (2003). Elder sexual abuse within the family. *Journal of Elder Abuse & Neglect, 15*(1), 43–58. doi:10.1300/J08-4v15n01_04

Ramsey-Klawsnik, H. (2007). Working with abuse perpetrators. *Victimization of the Elderly & Disabled, 10*(2), 19–20, 25.

Ramsey-Klawsnik, H. (2009). Elder sexual abuse. *National Association of Social Workers MA Chapter Focus Newsletter, 36*(4), 7–10, 15–17. (Available as an online continuing education course at www.naswma.org.)

Ramsey-Klawsnik, H., & Heisler, C. (2014). Polyvictimization in later life. *Victimization of the Elderly & Disabled, 17*(1), 3–4, 15–16.

Ramsey-Klawsnik, H. & Miller, E., (2017). Polyvictimization in later life: Trauma-informed best practices. *Journal of Elder Abuse & Neglect, 29*(5), 339–350. doi:10.1080/08946566.2017.1388017

Ramsey-Klawsnik, H., Teaster, P. B., Mendiondo, M. S., Marcum, J. L., & Abner, E. L. (2008). Sexual predators who target elders: Findings from the first national study of sexual abuse in care facilities. *Journal of Elder Abuse & Neglect, 20*(4), 353–376. doi:10.1080/08946560802359375

Rennison, C. M. (2001). *Intimate partner violence and age of victim, 1993–99* (NCJ 187635). Washington, DC: U.S. Department of Justice. Retrieved from http://www.ncjrs.gov/App/publications/Abstract.aspx?id=187635

Stonehouse, K., & Scahill, J. (2012). Finding her voice: An elder's triumph over communication barriers. *Victimization of the Elderly & Disabled, 15*(2), 17–18, 29–30.

Teaster, P. B., Dugar, T. A., Mendiondo, M. S., Abner, E. L., Cecil, K. A., & Otto, J. M. (2006). The 2004 Survey of State Adult Protective Services: Abuse of adults 60 years of age and older. Washington, DC: National Center on Elder Abuse. Retrieved from https://ncea.acl.gov/resources/docs/archive/APS-Adults-60plus-FactSheet-2006.pdf

Wolf, R. S. (2000). Introduction: The nature and scope of elder abuse. *Generations, 24*(2), 6–12.

Zink, T., Fisher, B. S., Regan, S., & Pabst, S. (2005). The prevalence and incidence of intimate partner violence in older women in primary care practices. *Journal of General Internal Medicine, 20*, 884–888. doi:10.1111/j.1525-1497.2005.0191.x

5

AMERICAN INDIAN PERSPECTIVES, CHALLENGES, AND APPROACHES TO ELDER ABUSE

Derrell W. Cox II and Lori L. Jervis

Chapter Objectives

By the end of this chapter, readers will be able to

1. Describe American Indian (AI) perspectives on elder abuse (EA).

2. Describe why and how the nexus of the EA of AIs is a public health issue.

3. Understand the current state of knowledge related to AIs and EA.

4. Explore how public health professionals can intervene in instances of the EA of AIs.

5. Understand the development of model codes, mandatory reporting, and outstanding programs that inform public health intervention and prevention efforts.

This chapter focuses on American Indian (AI) perspectives on elder abuse (EA)[1] and the unique challenges faced by these communities in dealing

---

[1] In this chapter, we use the terms "elder mistreatment" and "elder abuse" interchangeably, though we perceive mistreatment as being a broader and possibly more culturally appropriate term that includes financial exploitation, neglect, physical and psychological abuse, as well as disrespect (Jervis, Sconzert-Hall, & The Shielding American Indian Elders Project Team, 2017).

with this issue vis-à-vis their ongoing status as domestic-dependent nations (Maxwell & Maxwell, 1992). Although Native communities have often found themselves in a disadvantaged position with respect to dealing with the abuse, neglect, and financial exploitation of elders in their midst because of the lingering effects of colonialism, some tribes are developing approaches with greater relevance to their contemporary cultures.

As this chapter demonstrates, Native EA research and practice are relatively nascent fields. We attempt to highlight the current state of knowledge and practice in these communities and the importance of understanding indigenous perspectives and challenges regarding elder treatment. We begin with an overview of the major issues regarding EA in tribal communities, including a discussion of prevalence, risk factors, Native perspectives (with special attention given to one of the most common forms of elder mistreatment, financial exploitation), prevention strategies, policies at the federal and tribal levels, and jurisdictional concerns. The next section on "critical developments" examines development of model codes, mandatory reporting, and exemplary programs that discuss how strong connections can be formed between vulnerable elders, social services agencies, and police departments, as well as how multiple disciplines relate to each other to form effective research and response teams to address and prevent EA, especially the newly emerging field of study concerning an acutely toxic form of EA, polyvictimization. This section continues with ways to address and prevent incidents of abuse and its sequelae using policy and program frameworks based on alternative or traditional Native family- and community-centric values. These include family conferences, ombudsmen programs, sacred justice and restorative justice (RJ), and elder mediation. When abuse occurs, these models address abuse by identifying ways for offenders to provide restitution and be a part of the restoration of ruptured relationships, while ensuring the protection of vulnerable elders.

Finally, we look to future challenges and recommendations for those working with AI clients (including Adult Protective Services [APS] personnel) concerning ways that agencies can provide effective support for caregivers of elders. We then discuss briefly some of the differences between Western and traditional organizational procedures and models, and provide information about ways to enable culturally appropriate outreach to Native elders. Although we reference the larger U.S. Native population, which includes both AIs and Alaska Natives (ANs), the primary focus of this chapter is on AIs (defined here as those having origins in and maintaining an identification with the First Peoples of what is now the United States).

OVERVIEW OF ELDER ABUSE IN TRIBAL COMMUNITIES

Prevalence of Elder Abuse Among Tribes

To date, there have been no large-scale, population-based studies of the prevalence of EA among AIs; thus, EA prevalence among this population remains unknown (Jervis, 2014). A notable complicating obstacle to conducting prevalence studies among Natives is the diversity of this population, which includes 567 federally recognized AI tribes and AN villages (Bureau of Indian Affairs [BIA] & Cloud, 2016), each of which has its own culture and procedures for approving research conducted in its jurisdictions and communities. Nonetheless, it is possible to get a sense of the nature of elder mistreatment in smaller studies with nonrepresentative samples. Three studies in particular provide an indication of abuse in Native populations.

The first study was a survey of 110 "very traditional"[2] Navajo older adults and their families, followed by more detailed interviews of a small random sample of survey participants ($n = 37$). The researcher found that 16% of elders reported having experienced physical mistreatment (Brown, 1989). In a second study involving medical records review, Buchwald et al. (2000) found that 10% of 550 AI/AN) urban-residing patients at the Seattle Indian Health Board aged 50 years and older were definitely or probably abused in the past year. Where the gender of the abused was known, the majority (88.8%) were female, and their abusers were male (Buchwald et al., 2000). Abused individuals were more likely to be younger (the mean age of those who had experienced abuse was 56 years, whereas the mean age of those who had not experienced abuse was 62 years [Buchwald et al., 2000, p. 563]), female, experiencing depression, and dependent on others for food. Of those who were definitely abused, only 31% of cases had been reported to the authorities.

Somewhat differently, a community-based participatory research project that examined 100 urban and rural older AIs' perceptions of mistreatment by family found that 16% of participants stated that they had been treated badly by family members, whereas 76% discussed cases where other Native elders experienced such abuse (Jervis et al., 2017). Being exploited

---

[2] Brown (1989) describes "very traditional" as being geographically and culturally relatively isolated, primarily Navajo-speaking with little English spoken in homes, oriented primarily to Navajo cultural traditions, and subsisting pastorally with resource and responsibilities shared among extended family and clan networks (p. 20).

financially—for money (e.g., theft), labor (e.g., exploitative childcare), or housing—predominated in elders' reports, with neglect also an area of great concern. Substance abuse and culture loss were held responsible for much of the elder mistreatment within participants' communities.

Other studies give similar indications of the salience of neglect and financial exploitation in Native communities. In one study, neglect (32.4%) and financial exploitation (21.6%) were the most frequently reported types of abuse among Navajo elders (Brown, 1989). Neglect and financial exploitation were also the most common concerns on Lone Mountain, a remote, economically isolated, and resource-deprived reservation, whereas secondary neglect was the only form of elder mistreatment on the less isolated and relatively resource-adequate Abundant Lands reservation, which encompasses the entrance to a major U.S. national park and has a successful industry that employs local tribal members (Maxwell & Maxwell, 1992).

The extant research on Native elder mistreatment provides indications that the prevalence of elder physical mistreatment ranges between 10% and 16%. In the general population, however, it is believed that rates of reported physical abuse are just the "tip of the iceberg," far exceeded by emotional abuse, financial exploitation, and neglect (The National Center on Elder Abuse at The American Public Human Services Association & Westat Inc., 1998). In a national randomized survey of 5,777 older U.S. adults—of whom 2.3% ($n = 132$) identified as AI/AN—11.4% ($n = 589$) of the total sample had experienced at least one type of mistreatment in the previous year (Acierno et al., 2010; Acierno, as cited in Taylor, 2014). By type of mistreatment, the rates of past-year prevalence for the total sample ($n = 5,777$) were financial exploitation by a family member (5.2%, $n = 263$), potential neglect[3] (5.1%; $n = 297$), emotional mistreatment (4.6%; $n = 254$), physical mistreatment (1.6%; $n = 86$), and sexual mistreatment (0.6%; $n = 34$) (Acierno et al., 2010; Acierno, Hernandez-Tejado, Muzzy, & Steve, 2009). Thus, financial exploitation and neglect are more commonly reported than physical and sexual abuse from a national perspective. In addition, the reported rates of physical abuse in dedicated studies of Native communities are considerably higher than those found by Acierno (in one case, 10 times higher), though the various methodologies used by the respective studies no doubt strongly influenced their different findings. Also relevant, underreporting is certainly a possibility

---

[3] Potential neglect was defined as "an identified need for assistance that no one was actively addressing" (Acierno et al., 2010, p. 293).

in studies that use direct questioning methods due to social desirability bias, given the highly sensitive nature of elder mistreatment (de Jong, Pieters, & Fox, 2010).

Risk Factors

Similar to Pillemer's (1985) findings of risk factors for EA in the general U.S. population, Brown's (1989) surveys of elders and caregivers found that elder mistreatment in a small Navajo community was correlated with elder dependency (especially sudden-onset dependency), mental health concerns among both elders and their caregivers, and neglect because of caregiver fatigue or economic deprivation. Brown also found, like Maxwell and Maxwell (1992) in other reservation settings, that when an elder has an income, but lives with younger family members who are unemployed, the result is a Catch-22: Having an income made vulnerable elders more likely to experience psychological and physical abuse, while having no income or resources left elders more vulnerable to neglect (1989). In addition, Brown's findings pointed to increased risks for elder mistreatment when multiple persons shared caregiving responsibilities (1989); when everyone is responsible for care, no one is responsible (1989).

Brown, Fernandez, and Griffith (1990) asked 152 health and social service providers, law enforcement officers, tribal officials, and community volunteers about their views of the mistreatment of Navajo elders. These respondents indicated that victims were most commonly women, very old and physically vulnerable, socially isolated in their home, and perceived by their live-in caregivers as a burden (Brown, Fernandez, & Griffith, 1990). Typically, abusers were family caregivers with substance abuse issues and/or mental health issues such as depression who were unemployed, experiencing the effects of long-term poverty, and who took on the role of caregiving as yet another burden for which they did not have adequate resources (Brown et al., 1990).

More recent research has confirmed these earlier findings, with substantial evidence suggesting that for perpetrators, substance abuse, mental health problems, stress, history of child abuse, being overburdened, poor coping skills, and structural factors that engender hopelessness, poverty, and/or dependency on the elder are predictors of EA (Anisko, 2009; Smyer & Clark, 2011). For elders, being socially isolated, having mental health issues, chronic illness, stress, and being dependent on the perpetrator are associated with experiencing abuse from their caregiver (Anisko, 2009; Smyer & Clark, 2011).

RESEARCH BOX

The Impact of Systemic and Structural Factors on Native Elder Abuse

Maxwell and Maxwell's (1992) important archival research, ethnographic work, and sociological analyses among two different Northern Plains tribes use a historical and political ecological approach to frame the different prevalence of EA they found between the pseudonymic Lone Mountain tribe (a small, rural, and geographically isolated community with no industrial development, tourist attractions, and inadequate agricultural resources) and the also pseudonymic Abundant Lands tribe (whose lands are situated in close proximity to a national park and through which visitors must pass, resulting in abundant opportunities for economic development and commerce). Both tribes were of similar economic and subsistence styles at early contact with Euro-Americans and have experienced similar culturally disintegrating pressures through assimilation policies, such as boarding schools, missionary religious reeducation, and Indian agencies that forced AI tribal members to comply with Euro-American lifeways or starve. Nevertheless, by the time of Maxwell and Maxwell's research in 1988, there were major differences in the living conditions, socioeconomic status, and prevalence of EA between the tribes (1992). These differing conditions were primarily driven by structural and systemic factors outside of the control of either tribe or its members, though different responses to economic assimilation pressures by each tribe contributed in smaller ways (1992). In sum, the socioeconomic advantages available to residents of the Abundant Lands reservation allow the younger generations to remain integrated into sustainable communities, which ultimately reduced risks for abuse and neglect of elders. The isolation, socioeconomic disadvantages, and inadequate agricultural resources of the Lone Mountain reservation drove away younger generations with abilities to earn wages off of the reservation. Those remaining had fewer options and often subsisted as adult dependents of the elders who controlled what resources and lands were available. This, theoretically, resulted in higher rates of elder mistreatment, including physical and emotional abuse and neglect (1992).

Maxwell and Maxwell (1992) were careful to emphasize that even on Lone Mountain, the majority of intergenerational relationships were "cooperative and often warm" (p. 6). Nonetheless, their insight that

(continued)

structural factors can play a large role in interpersonal relationships was an important one. In the case of Indian country, when mistreatment does occur, it does so in the postcolonial cultural context that in too many tribal settings includes "pervasive poverty, dislocation, diminished health, and overcrowded tribal housing" (Jervis, 2014; see also Buchwald et al., 2000; Maxwell & Maxwell, 1992; Nerenberg, 1999; Nerenberg et al., 2004b; Walsh et al., 2010). It may also co-occur in homes with child maltreatment and intimate partner violence.

Native Understandings of Abuse

Despite cultural variability among tribal groups, the vast majority of tribal members would likely agree that respect for elders is an important value within their culture. In addition, there is a wide degree of latitude concerning what constitutes culturally acceptable behavior toward older adults across cultures worldwide, on a continuum from eldercide of those who are believed to have become a burden to the community on one end to loving care and veneration on the other, sometimes varying with the physical and mental frailty or strength of the elder (Barker, 2009; Coon, 1948; Glascock, 2009; Gray & Gregor, 1878; Maxwell & Maxwell, 1992). Each cultural group holds different ideals and perceptions of appropriate eldercare as well as what constitutes mistreatment (Jervis, 2014; Jervis et al., 2017; Rittman, Kuzmeskus, & Flum, 1999). Actions perceived by one cultural group as abusive may not be regarded as abusive by another, whereas actions seen as nonabusive in one group may be regarded as abusive in another (Hudson, Armachain, Beasley, & Carlson, 1998; Hudson & Carlson, 1999; Jervis, 2014).

For example, research with 424 White, 318 African American, and 202 Native American adults ($N = 944$) aged 40 years and older residing in North Carolina found similar perceptions of what constitutes elder mistreatment across all three groups based on their responses to 26 questions pertaining to elder mistreatment (Hudson et al., 1998; Hudson & Carlson, 1999). These similar perceptions of mistreatment included "assault; battery; threatening; coercion; unreasonable confinement, intimidation, or cruelty; sexual abuse; emotional abuse; intimidation; exploitation, abandonment; and breach of fiduciary duty" (Hudson et al., 1998; Hudson & Carlson, 1999). However, Native elders were more likely to categorize a case study as abuse, to deem a single incident as abuse, and to consider an incident severe than were the other ethnic groups (Brown, 1989; Hudson et al., 1998; Hudson & Carlson, 1999).

In a study of elder mistreatment among 100 older AIs, good treatment was conceived of in terms of being taken care of, having one's needs met, and being respected (Jervis et al., 2017). Elders maintained relatively high standards for how they should be treated by family members (e.g., the notion that an elder's needs should be anticipated and met without the elder needing to ask). Poor treatment primarily consisted of financial exploitation and neglect, with lack of respect, psychological abuse, and physical abuse also described. This research also identified gray areas, such as exploitative childcare (Jervis, 2014; Jervis et al., 2017). For example, although elders reported feeling disrespected when grandchildren were nonconsensually left in their care, culturally normative close grandchild–grandparent relationships involving both child care by the grandparent and eldercare by the grandchild (Jervis, Boland, & Fickenscher, 2010; Schweitzer, 1999) blur the lines between exploitation and culturally acceptable behavior. This situation can make it difficult for communities to ascertain when "lines are being crossed," especially Native elders who are not sure to what extent they are "being disrespected" (Jervis, 2014; Jervis, Fickenscher, Beals, & Shielding AI Elders Project Team, 2014; Jervis et al., 2017). The lines between exploitation and culturally appropriate sharing are also blurred where the sharing of money and other material resources are concerned.

Financial Exploitation

The issue of financial exploitation in Native communities is complex. Many tribal groups maintain within-group systems of reciprocity while using mainstream economic systems with outsiders (Pickering, 2000). Thus, within their local communities, an elder's sharing of resources with family members has been historically (and remains presently) a "cultural privilege and duty" for the elder (Brown, 1989; Smyer & Clark, 2011). In some cases, caring for elders within Native contexts may be understood as a source of fulfillment to both caregivers and care recipients, rather than as a burden (Carson, 1995; Carson & Hand, 1999; Jervis et al., 2010; Smyer & Clark, 2011). Historically, traditional socioeconomic systems of reciprocity, such as giveaways and other resource distribution rituals, functioned to reequalize society, confer honor to the givers, maintain equilibrium in spiritual domains, and, on the whole, maintain social cohesion and familial and economic interdependency (Cole & Chaikin, 1990; Moore, 1996; Red Horse, 1983; Smyer & Clark, 2011). These and other community-building customs brought opposition from U.S. federal colonizing forces, who valued individualism, land ownership, and capitalism

as the pathway to "civilization" (Dawes, 1886; Harmon, 2003). These colonizing forces systematically overwhelmed, displaced, and disrupted traditional
lifeways, gender roles, kinship systems, and land-usage patterns, which in turn
negatively altered the ways that elders were treated (Biolsi, 1992; Cattelino,
2008; Jervis & the AI-SUPERPFP Team, 2009; Jervis, Spicer, Manson, & the
AI-SUPERPFP Team, 2003; Maxwell & Maxwell, 1992; Nerenberg, Baldridge,
& Benson, 2004b; Pickering, 2000; Prucha, 1978; Sturm, 2002; Walsh, Olson,
Ploeg, Lohfeld, & MacMillan, 2010; White, 2004). For example, where the
locus of spiritual, moral, and subsistence resources once flowed from the
elders (some of whom were chiefs and healers) to the community—a process that validated their authority, enabled them to fulfill their responsibility to oversee the community's welfare, and established a firm basis for
elder respect—colonial policies replaced these traditional lines of authority
with individuals willing to function within colonial government mandates
(e.g., see Biolsi, 1992). This paved the way for assimilation, but also stripped
the elders and traditional leadership of the resources, respect, and moral
authority to lead. In disrupting normative age expectations, colonialism
effectively reduced some older citizens who in times past would have been
highly esteemed to a state of vulnerability and dependence, effectively
setting them up for abuse (Biolsi, 1992; Fowler, 2004; Hudson et al., 1998;
Knack, 2004; Maxwell & Maxwell, 1992).

This is not to suggest that elders cannot be financially exploited within
economic systems in which reciprocity is highly valued—indeed, they can be
and are. Financial exploitation may be an especially common form of elder
mistreatment among some Native communities, as it is among the general
population (Acierno et al., 2010; Brown et al., 1990; Jervis et al., 2017; Maxwell & Maxwell, 1992; Nerenberg, Baldridge, & Benson, 2004a). In societies where reciprocity is expected, an unemployed adult child or grandchild
may pressure the elder to provide economic assistance, placing the elder
in a dilemma of either contributing to the needs of others or meeting the
elder's own immediate needs (e.g., medicine or food). Contributing to the
support of kin in need may be viewed as an obligation of an extended family
member that cannot be neglected if one has ever had or might in the future
require such support from one's kin group. Making sense of this disjunc-
ture between traditional values that stress community and intergenerational
reciprocity and a more recent reality where that reciprocal relationship is
violated (often by the same children and grandchildren who provide care) is
a challenge for contemporary Native communities.

An aspect of mistreatment that has received a fair amount of attention among Native elders, but that is not often considered by the dominant

society, is spiritual abuse, defined as "the erosion or breaking down of one's cultural or religious belief system" (Malley-Morrison & Hines, 2004, p. 62; Marshall & Vaillancourt, 1993, p. 155). Spiritual abuse may include behavior such as being denied access to ceremonies, traditional healing, or healers or having traditional regalia taken without permission. Spiritual abuse prevents Native elders from connecting with their cultural, spiritual, and language traditions (Dumont-Smith & Aboriginal Healing Foundation, 2002; Nerenberg et al., 2004a). The ability for an elder to teach others is also crucial, as this teaching ensures the continuity of tribal and spiritual values from past generations into the present and onward to future generations (Crowshoe & Manneschmidt, 2002; Mails & Crow, 1979; Powers, 1986; Smyer & Clark, 2011).

Elder Abuse Case Study 1

Spiritual Abuse

The following is a composite (to deidentify subjects) of two AI elders' accounts of spiritual abuse (though they both experienced polyvictimization) as told to and/or observed by the lead author. All names are pseudonymic.

Ruth was 70 years old and in the final stages of terminal cancer. She lived with and received hospice care from her daughter, Elsie, and Elsie's family in an urban location two hours from her home on the reservation. Ruth retired 10 years ago and returned to live on the reservation where she was born and raised. Her cultural values have always been important to her, and they have grown increasingly important as she aged. During a hospital stay, a conflict between Ruth and Elsie (who identifies as an evangelical Christian) over Ruth's request to have a traditional healer perform a ceremony in the hospital resulted in minor damage to hospital property (broken coffee cup and saucer, damage to a clothing wardrobe) when Ruth's daughter threw a tray of food in anger during the conflict. Ruth's friend's appeal to the hospital staff to permit a traditional healer to visit during Elsie's absence was then rejected because of hospital policy. Ruth felt demoralized by Elsie's refusal to permit the traditional healer to come first to the hospital and then to the home during what she believes are her final days on earth.

In their study, Maxwell and Maxwell (1992) described the perspectives of two Northern Plains tribes where elder mistreatment is presented as being the result of a breach in the health of the community as a whole, which requires community-wide solutions. Mistreatment toward an elder is an insult that transcends the elder's body and damages the integrity of the community as a whole (Maxwell & Maxwell, 1992; Red Horse, 1980, 1983, 1997). Such a notion contrasts with what some tribal members and communities see as commonly held beliefs of the dominant culture that mistreatment is a private matter involving only individuals and some family members, requiring punitive, individual- or family-level sanctions (Forer, 1994; Maxwell & Maxwell, 1992). The community-level focus found in these examples echoes the previous calls by Baker (1975), Butler (1975), and Burston (1975) for elder mistreatment to be understood as a public health issue that requires structural as well as community- and individual-level solutions. Rather than focusing only on the malicious actions of an individual perpetrator, many Native communities are keenly interested in rooting mistreatment in community- and structural-level dysfunction. This dysfunction takes into account the impact of colonization and the subsequent loss of homelands, which brought with it a lack of essential resources for sociocultural and economic subsistence, combined with steep gradients of inequality that have continued since the 19th century (Maxwell & Maxwell, 1992; Brave Heart, 2003). Although individual dysfunction may be psychologized and criminalized, by being cast into the realm of community dysfunction, elder mistreatment is politicized.

Elder Abuse Case Study 2

Polyvictimization and Abuse Escalation

This case is a composite of several elders encountered in a variety of research projects and contacts with Native communities.

Native elders often experience multiple forms of mistreatment. Sandy, an older AI woman living in a rural setting, had six grown children, one of whom (Sam) struggled with a serious case of substance abuse. Over the years, this son's life began to fall apart and Sandy took him in. Sam began to have parties at her house that lasted late into the night, severely stressing her out and making her feel disrespected. Sam's requests for financial help soon became

(continued)

Elder Abuse Case Study 2 (*continued*)

demands; if Sandy did not supply him with money, her possessions or medications (especially prescription painkillers) would go missing. Early on, Sandy comforted herself with the thought that her son was "only a heavy drinker" who was never "violent," but he eventually began insulting her while drunk, claiming that she had not been "there for him" while he was growing up. Sandy believed she deserved these "tongue lashings" because she herself had a drinking problem when the kids were growing up. Eventually, however, the tongue lashings took on a more threatening feel and Sam began to put holes in the wall. During one argument, Sandy happened to be standing in front of Sam trying to calm him down when his fist found her face. Sam began to cry, saying he didn't mean for it to happen. Realizing he was intoxicated, Sandy forgave him. However, as Sam's substance abuse escalated, the physical abuse eventually became a pattern, with Sandy hiding it from her other children, terrified that Sam would be put into prison and that the family would be "broken up."

In summary, although exact prevalence figures are hard to come by for Native groups, EA is generally considered problematic; the proper arena for dealing with abuse is not necessarily confined to individuals and dyads. In response, tribal entities have enacted policies and response strategies to define and prevent EA as well as to call those who mistreat to account.

Prevention and Policy

The Older Americans Act of 1965 (OAA; see also Chapter 3) was passed in U.S. Congress and signed into law to address national concerns about the health and well-being of U.S. Americans aged 60 and older. Title VII of OAA provided funds for states to create programs to provide protection for vulnerable elders. Title IV and Title VI of the OAA specifically addressed some of the unique needs of Native American elders and provided funding for program development for their support in the areas of (a) establishing resource centers that gather information; (b) conducting and disseminating results of research; (c) providing technical assistance and training, especially in the areas of health, mental health, long-term care, EA, and other concerns;

(d) nutrition services or meal programs; (e) funding for improving or altering multipurpose senior centers; (f) legal services; and (g) other supports. Despite the many benefits that came with the OAA, some felt that culturally appropriate provision of services were not adequately ensured by this law (Nerenberg et al., 2004a, 2004b)

Nearly two decades would transpire before culturally appropriate guidelines or laws were developed through the reauthorization of the OAA to define, prevent, and remediate elder mistreatment by tribal communities themselves, first by the Oglala Lakota Nation in 1984, then by the Yakima Nation a few years later (National Center on Elder Abuse, 1995; Oglala Sioux Tribe, 2002 [1984]; Yakima Indian Nation, 1987). Several more years passed before studies began to be conducted examining elder mistreatment in tribal communities (Brown, 1989; Brown et al., 1990; Maxwell & Maxwell, 1992; U.S. Senate Resolution 88-14, 1988). Within a few years of these seminal studies on elder mistreatment in tribal communities, AIs, ANs, and First Nations of Canada began to assemble to address this issue within their communities (National Association of State Units on Aging 1989; Nerenberg et al., 2004a).

The National Indian Council on Aging, an advocacy organization for tribal elders, provides a number of useful guidelines for tribes and supporting agencies as they develop and implement policies and programs for preventing, intervening, and addressing elder mistreatment (Nerenberg et al., 2004b). Undergirding these guidelines is the belief that tribally specific traditional values and beliefs should inform, reflect, and provide the basis for programs from conception through design and implementation to evaluation. Community consensus-building and intergenerational dialogue should determine culturally appropriate programs and policies that will

> promote family unity and cooperation; reflect traditional models of dispute resolution; employ informal community networks; [and] attempt to prevent abuse by maintaining or supporting families and preserving and restoring cultural values and traditions. (Nerenberg et al., 2004b, p. 6)

In addition, these programs and policies must recognize and respect tribal sovereignty, including the nature and extent of the tribe's involvement and control over EA prevention and justice programs, as well as how the tribal and nontribal agencies cooperate and interrelate. Programs and policies must be specifically tailored to each tribe, allowing for their own unique histories and traditions regarding interpersonal and community disruptions to be processed and addressed (Jackson & Sappier, 2005; Nerenberg et al., 2004a, 2004b). These may include multiple areas of traditional jurisdictions over the care and protection of elders, including the family and extended family, tribal elders and healers, peacemakers and mediators, and tribal courts, in addition to tribal and nontribal social and government agencies and legal systems. It is important that tribal, local, state, and federal agencies, along with state and federal governments, mitigate or eradicate structural factors that increase the likelihood of abuse and neglect of elders, such as high rates of youth and young adult unemployment, inadequate or nonexistent funding for culturally appropriate childcare and eldercare, and lack of culturally appropriate nutrition assistance programs that recognize the multigenerational households commonly encountered in AI communities. Appropriately addressing these factors will undermine core drivers of abuse (Nerenberg et al., 2004b).

Jurisdictional Issues and Tribal Law and Order Act of 2010

One of the most significant challenges facing Native communities with respect to EA has been the lack of a tribal legal framework with which to respond. Without a framework that empowers tribes to respond to crime that approximates what is taken for granted by other U.S. citizens, it is difficult for tribes to move toward more sophisticated legal and public health programs and interventions. To date, fewer than 10% of the United States' 567 federally recognized tribes and Alaskan Native Villages have developed EA codes. These tribes may legislate sanctions against EA under criminal or civil codes, depending on its severity.

With the passage of the Tribal Law and Order Act of 2010 (TLOA), all tribes have the opportunity to revise their tribal codes to benefit from the opportunities encoded in the act. The TLOA results in more formalized processes within tribal courts, but permits them to mandate longer sentences, which are especially needed in the case of more serious crimes. It permits tribes to prosecute violations and establish sentences of one year or more in jail and to prosecute non-Native offenders for offenses committed within tribal jurisdictional areas. Although the TLOA provides many advantages for tribes, without adequate funding sources, under-resourced tribes frequently are unable to bear the additional costs associated with fulfilling their responsibilities under the act, such as appointing and funding a legally qualified judge, prosecutor, and public defender.

EA in Indian country has frequently gone unaddressed as a result of jurisdictional barriers that cross tribal, state, and federal geographic and legal boundaries in terms of which laws or codes have been violated and in which venue these charges will be prosecuted. The TLOA recognized the inadequacy of existing law enforcement resources within tribal lands and provided for training of tribal law and order personnel, cross-deputizing of law enforcement entities, and sharing of resources among tribal, federal, state, county, and local agencies so that laws may be enforced across jurisdictional boundaries. The TLOA also provides the framework to establish a memorandum of understanding (MOU) between tribes and local, county, and/ or state agencies concerning these shared resources and cooperative efforts. It provides that cases occurring in tribal and nontribal jurisdictions may be prosecuted concurrently by all relevant jurisdictions (TLOA, Subtitle B, Section 401, a (2)) It also provides for the prosecution of non-Indians who commit crimes on Indian lands, which, except for federal offenses, had not been possible earlier. Thus, in an area where a tribe has an MOU with federal, state, county, or local governments regarding the investigation, arrest, and prosecution of offenders, in the financial exploitation scenario mentioned earlier, the MOU would allow the state-chartered bank to cooperate with the tribal officials by providing evidence concerning deposits and withdrawals by the caregiver, allowing tribal law enforcement to arrest, and a tribal court to prosecute, the caregiver (whether a tribal member or a non-Indian).

The TLOA allows tribes that have adequate resources and qualified legal staff to prosecute perpetrators of EA and to sentence for more than one year. As such, it provides greater legal parity between AI communities and the rest of the United States, contributes to public health goals by establishing the perception that legal justice is possible, and potentially separates perpetrators from their victims for the duration of their sentences. We argue that a functioning justice system is essential for individuals and communities to feel and actually be safe, which is essential to both physical and mental health.

In sum, the TLOA allows local, county, state, tribal, and federal officials to work together for the enforcement of laws across jurisdictions regardless of whether the perpetrators or victims are Indian or non-Indian. The TLOA presents an opportunity for tribes to initiate prosecutions and exercise their sovereignty in ways beneficial to their people, rather than waiting passively for state or federal agencies to act (Cross, 2014). As such, the TLOA provides greater flexibility for tribes, government officials and agencies, and public health staff to more effectively respond to EA at local, tribal, state, and national levels.

CRITICAL DEVELOPMENTS, PROMISING PRACTICES, AND REMAINING CHALLENGES

Development of Model Codes

Although EA model codes have been available through the Southern Plains Tribal Law Center, the Tribal Law and Policy Institute, and other organizations, fewer than 50 tribes to date have EA codes in their tribal law (National Indigenous Elder Justice Initiative [NIEJI], 2017). Development of a model tribal code for EA that is in compliance with the TLOA is difficult because of several factors, including the cultural and historical diversity of the 567 federally recognized tribal entities and AN villages in the United States; existing codes addressing EA that may be disbursed throughout various tribal codes (e.g., family, health and safety, and criminal sections), making a unified and single location within tribal codes a complex legislative process; and tribes covered and affected by Public Law 83-280 (PL 280), which require special attention, such as the need to establish civil codes for minor infractions (often by a family member and/or minor property theft) and criminal codes for incidents of severe abuse that would be prosecuted in criminal courts (TLOA of 2010, 2010). PL 280, enacted in 1953, transferred significant civil and criminal legal jurisdiction over tribal lands from the federal government to five—then six—U.S. states (California, Wisconsin, Minnesota, Nebraska, Oregon, and, upon statehood, Alaska). Since its enactment, other states have joined, whereas some tribes have withdrawn from this jurisdiction (Public Law 280, 1953). PL 280 tribes have compacts with the states where their lands and facilities are situated to use state resources for EA reporting, investigation, and prosecution. Correspondingly, PL 280 tribes benefit from state jurisdiction over non-Indians and cooperation in bringing offenders to justice; PL 280 tribes also benefit from additional state resources for the prosecution and investigation of civil and criminal matters, unlike non-PL 280 tribes that have no such agreements.

Mandatory Reporting

Although mandatory reporting laws require that people in certain professions (e.g., healthcare and social work) report suspected EA to an investigating authority, mandatory reporting is believed to be uncommon within many AI tribes. Outside formal contexts with required mandatory reporting, there is evidence that people are often very reluctant to report abuse for a variety of reasons, especially among cultures that value familial and kinship cohesiveness more than the rights or health of any individual member (Beaulaurier, Seff, Newman, & Dunlop, 2005). These reasons may include the elder's dependency on the abuser for assistance (economic, shelter, and general care) and the major disruption and heightened vulnerability that would occur in inadequate resource settings by causing harm to the abusive caregiver, as well as shame about failures to act in accordance with tribal expectations and cultural values concerning respect for elders (Anisko, 2009; Carson & Hand, 1999; Smyer & Clark, 2011; Walsh et al., 2010). Another reason may be the elder's awareness of his or her geographic isolation from social services and police, which are already understaffed and yet responsible for serving large reservation and rural areas, coupled with the high likelihood of repeated contact with the perpetrator after reporting abuse. Finally, there may be reticence to report because of the shame and humiliation that reporting would bring upon the elder and his or her family and distrust of law enforcement and federal agents (Anisko, 2009; Carson & Hand, 1999; Jervis, 2014; Nerenberg et al., 2004b; Shipler, Anand, & Hadi, 1998; Smyer & Clark, 2011; Wakeling, Jorgensen, Michaelson, & Begay, 2001). In addition, there is the very real concern that the punitive aspect of the justice system may do more harm than good in the long term. One elder remarked, "Jail doesn't help anyone. A lot of our people could have been healed a long time ago if it weren't for jail. Jail hurts them more, and then they come out really bitter. In jail all they learn is hurt and bitterness" (Nerenberg et al., 2004b, p. 30).

In summary, elders who experience mistreatment must assess the costs versus the benefits of reporting the incidents to police or agencies that may be associated with colonizing forces or contemporary ineffectiveness. For many, the results of these analyses force them to choose the lesser of "two evils"—which may be tolerating physical, emotional, financial, or sexual harm or neglect rather than subjecting themselves and their families to greater harm from other sources, such as deeper poverty, fewer resources, homelessness, unfamiliar environments (e.g., nursing homes far from their tribal lands and communities), and increased vulnerability and desperation (Beaulaurier et al., 2005; Beaulaurier, Seff, Newman, & Dunlop, 2007). Because only a small number of tribes have nursing homes, if an elder's caregivers are subjected to prosecution and are barred from the home, and if the elder has no other viable means of care or residence, then placement in a nursing home will usually be at a significant distance from the elder's home, far removed from family and friends. This is inconsistent with the sociocultural norms of eldercare by family members, both close and extended, found within many AI contexts (Hennessy & John, 1996; Litton & Ybanez, 2015).

Exemplary Programs

We now examine exceptional and promising programs and innovations to address and prevent EA from the areas of justice, policy development, and intervention within Indian country, involving several disciplines—namely, social services, law enforcement, medicine, jurisprudence, nursing, and tribal, state, and federal governments.

An exemplary model initiated by some tribes and tribal agencies has focused on the early detection of EA. For example, in Anadarko, Oklahoma (the historical and/or bureaucratic home of the Kiowa Nation, Comanche Nation, Apache Tribe, Wichita and Affiliated Tribes, Caddo Nation, Delaware Nation, and Fort Sill Apache Tribe), community agencies work to safeguard and encourage vulnerable elders. The Anadarko Agency Branch of Social Services' "Operation Golden Shield Project" provides an updated name and address list of vulnerable elders to Agency police, who conduct periodic social visits with vulnerable elders (Allen, Longhat, & Melton, 2013). As part of a program originally conceived by Rick Decora, former Chief of Police for the Anadarko Agency, police officers conduct random visits with three or four of more than 50 community-dwelling, vulnerable elders to check on their well-being and assess for indicators of physical, psychological, or financial abuse (Allen et al., 2013). Operation Golden Shield fosters positive, trusting relationships between these vulnerable elders and police officers, and also provides an opportunity for these elders to have safe social interaction. This ongoing collaboration has also implemented social and protective outreach programs for vulnerable elders, such as distribution of refrigerator magnets with important contact information about BIA services, periodic meal distribution, and Golden Angel and Golden Sweetheart gift programs that enlist community support and contributions for vulnerable elders during the Christmas season and Valentine's Day (Allen et al., 2013).

Multidisciplinary Teams and Elder Protection Teams

EA and prevention multidisciplinary teams (MDTs) may be developed within tribal communities to use the expertise and knowledge of locally available services for elders in the community, which may include an MDT coordinator, law enforcement, social services, courts, attorneys, counselors, fiduciaries, caregivers, health providers, BIA personnel, Federal Bureau of Investigation personnel, and APS from tribes, states, and/or counties (Jackson & DOJ, 2016 [2015]). There are several types of MDTs, which are uniquely developed to address local community needs and available staffing and resources. These MDTs may be drawn from resources within, including tribes, Public Law 280 states/tribes, multi/intertribal councils (e.g., some or all the tribes within a geographic area, state, or affiliated culture group may share resources and/or personnel, such as a tribal ombudsman, where resources are limited to provide better services to all member tribes), states, and federal agencies. MDTs all work in much the same way to assess areas of risk and needs, and to pursue justice for vulnerable adults. Effective MDTs include shared decision making, clearly defined partnership roles through MOUs or interagency agreements, interdependency in collaboration, balanced power so that no member or agency dominates the group, and clearly defined protocols to provide predictability, accountability, and conflict resolution—all for the purpose of improving care and treatment of older adults (Jackson & DOJ, 2016 [2015]). In such settings, caregivers may be provided with knowledge, training, and resources to improve their capacity for compassionate care. They may also experience subtle and not so subtle forms of accountability, as they are aware that their actions are being monitored by multiple individuals and agencies, which may serve to discourage future abuse, neglect, or exploitation.

MDTs may be useful in addressing one "wicked problem" (Churchman, 1967; Rittel & Webber, 1973) faced by elder adults, termed polyvictimization (Heisler, 2017; Teaster, 2017). Polyvictimization is when vulnerable elders experience multiple forms of concurrent abuse or repeated acts of the same abuse that are exacerbated over time, whether by one or more perpetrators (Ramsey-Klawsnik et al., 2014). Polyvictimization is a better predictor of physical and mental health status than any single abusive event (Hamby, Smith, Mitchell, & Turner, 2016). As in other forms of EA, and though there are significant vice versa cases, victims tend to be females and perpetrators are more often males, who range from teenagers to very old age (Roberto, 2017). Likewise, perpetrators frequently have histories of substance or alcohol abuse, have mental health issues, are often unemployed and/or dependent on the elder they abuse, frequently are related to the victim, and may cultivate trusting relationships with their victims, before beginning to exploit, coerce, or abuse them (Roberto, 2017). Polyvicitimization in later life has only recently emerged as a focus of study. It is complex and multifaceted, and stems from issues in the microsocial and macrosocial domains (Teaster, 2017). It is recommended that polyvictimization be prioritized for further research and investigation (Heisler, 2017; Roberto, 2017; Teaster, 2017).

Family Conference

The Family Care Conference is an elder-focused, family-centered intervention for preventing and mitigating elder mistreatment that uses trained community members as group facilitators (Holkup, Salois, Tripp-Reimer, & Weinert, 2007; Salois, Holkup, Tripp-Reimer, & Weinert, 2006). On the basis of a model developed by the Maori in New Zealand, this model has been used extensively by U.S. states and other nations in intervening in child maltreatment, but has not been systematically applied to elder protection. The Family Care Conference consists of six processes or phases: referrals, screening, engagement with family, logistical preparation, the family meeting, and follow-up. This model was piloted in one northwestern Native American community using a community-based participatory research strategy (Salois et al., 2006). Results while the study was ongoing showed that families appreciated the Family Care Conference's emphasis on bringing the family into harmony and finding solutions within the family and community (Holkup et al., 2007). Thus, this model shows promise as another alternative to dealing with EA in Indian country, especially in cases where abuse or neglect does not appear to be life-threatening.

Ombudsman Programs

The Administration on Aging/Administration on Community Living (AoA/ACL) asserts that Tribal Long-Term Care Ombudsman programs are effective resources for ensuring quality of care in long-term care facilities (Hollister & Estes, 2013). The ombudsman position enables the tribal system to comply with the TLOA. An ombudsman hears and investigates complaints between parties prior to involving legal or human services in an investigation of EA. Concerned parties can go to the ombudsman and request an inquiry into the issue at hand, and the ombudsman will then advise, mediate, or assist in making referrals to other services. Long-Term Care Ombudsman Programs do not provide services to elders who reside in their own homes or those of relatives. Additional resources would be necessary for ombudsmen to address EA issues in community settings outside of nursing homes (Hollister & Estes, 2013). If ombudsman services were available through elder services provided by tribal programs to these elders residing in their own homes or with family, it might provide a beneficial intermediary where other, more comprehensive services are unavailable. The tribal or intertribal council ombudsman could either act in the elder's behalf or serve as an advocate for finding needed resources.

POLICY BOX

Reporting Abuse in Reservation Communities

Native elders and fellow community members in reservation communities are sometimes hesitant to report abuse because of a conviction that the system will be unresponsive and that they or family members may face retribution; fear that the perpetrator will be arrested—and that the elder's grandchildren will end up in (possibly non-Native) foster care; or fear in situations where either the elder or the perpetrator is in the role of caregiver that a report of abuse could lead to institutionalization in a distant nursing home. In these circumstances, those who are concerned about elder mistreatment are left with few good options. An important question is which policy changes are required for both elders and community members to feel safe in reporting cases of abuse, and which resources are needed to make abuse reporting safe and effective in improving outcomes.

Alternatives to the Legal System

The term "sacred justice" refers to processes for resolving interpersonal and community conflicts used in many traditional tribal contexts that are becoming more commonplace in tribal programs (LeResche, 1993). Sacred justice reflects tribal values and practices by focusing on the restoration of balance within relationships, rather than on the retributive justice (where the primary goal is to punish, rather than rehabilitate, the offender) or distributive justice (which focuses on equitable distribution of resources) used in U.S. judicial systems (LeResche, 1993). Similar processes used within Native contexts, such as RJ, peacemaker programs, elder councils, and family meetings, focus on restoration of relationships, social equilibrium, and healing for both offended and offender rather than retributive justice (LeResche, 1993).

RJ is based on a conceptual framework that recognizes offenses as damaging to not only victims but also the families of the offender(s), victim(s), and community as a whole. Primarily, RJ considers abuse as a violation of people and relationships, rather than a violation of the law. RJ establishes goals of understanding of criminogenesis and the etiology of biopsychosocial pathologies to prevent future offenses and offenders/perpetrators, restitution

of damages (where possible) by the offender, restoration of relationships ruptured by the offense, and healing from traumas experienced by both victims
and offenders to reestablish harmony, trust, and safety within the community.

Elder mediation has similar end goals to RJ, but with a mediation-
focused process to bring together all affected persons to find solutions that
are mutually agreeable. Peacemaking, a form of sacred justice, contrasts with
Anglo-American justice, drawing from indigenous cultural values of healing and healers, restitution, and restoration of affected relationships when
practicable, and working toward social equilibrium in the present and future
through ceremonies in community and family contexts, rather than focusing on judges, judgment, punishment, past wrongs, and attribution of guilt
and shame within courtrooms (Wolf, 2012a, 2012b).

In contrast to policies enforced by the dominant society that are imposed
upon Native peoples (Carson & Hand, 1999; Gordon, 1988, 1994), AI/AN
communities are argued to comprise centuries-old, deeply interconnected
"communities of relatedness" that have endured across generations in spite
of the dominant society's relatively recently formed "collectivities of strangers" and their attempts to assimilate or eradicate AI/AN communities (Hand,
1996). When "communities of relatedness" seek to address behaviors and
actions of those within their society, it is done with the ultimate goal of
restoring peace and right relations within the community, which makes
RJ models well suited for Native contexts. RJ calls upon individuals within
society to advocate for and commit to humane and socially just policies
that ultimately provide healing to victims and restore offenders into healthy
relationships within healthy societies (Elliott, 2011). RJ models emerging in
North America have come out of the First Nations of Canada and are now
being adopted by various tribes in North America (Haslip, 2002), as well as
non-Native communities.

As it pertains to elder mistreatment specifically, RJ is a mechanism for
bringing together the elder, abuser(s), caregiver(s), and other family and
community members of both victim and perpetrator to look for a positive
approach and long-term solution for all involved without involving the
courts (Elliott, 2011; Ellis, 2009; National Institute of Justice, 2007; Umbreit,
1989; van Ness, 1990). There is usually a written plan that the parties agree
to and that outlines what the consequences will be if the plan is not followed.
This is a preferred approach when the EA or neglect was perpetrated by a
family member whom the elder does not want to see prosecuted and sent
to jail, hence making him or her reluctant to take action should there be future violations. In cases where caregiver stress is a contributing factor and
where respite can be arranged, RJ can have a very positive result. However, in

---

DISCUSSION BOX

Western and Native-Based Approaches to Criminal Justice in Indian Country

In this chapter, you have been presented with alternatives to the Western criminal justice system when working with Native EA, including promoting healing and mediation approaches as alternatives to the court system.

1. Do you find these alternatives promising? Do you think these alternatives apply only to Native communities or extend beyond them?

2. How much of the problem within the Western justice system in Native communities might relate to its ineffective or incomplete implementation or lack of resources?

3. Perhaps the problem is primarily poor cultural fit. What do you think about some of the alternative approaches emerging in Native communities that are described here (e.g., programs to strengthen connections between vulnerable elders and police/social services; spiritual justice; family conferences)? Are these approaches culturally specific (i.e., only applicable to Native communities), or might they be more widely used?

---

cases involving substance abuse and/or severe physical abuse, RJ may not be a viable alternative.

THE FUTURE: ISSUES TO BE RESOLVED

Challenges

An issue discussed anecdotally among those working in Native communities is that of the nonrecognition of elder mistreatment, primarily among elders but also among tribal leaders and those poised to make a difference in this area (BigFoot et al., 2000; Nerenberg et al., 2004b). Without recognition of the problem—and the will to make a change—the likelihood that EA will be reported or that new programs will be put into place is greatly diminished. Stretched resources in some tribes, combined with a focus on the issues that concern young people (who are demographically much more numerous in Native populations),[4] are explanations for a lack of political will, as is ageism (Nahmiash, 2004; Walsh et al., 2010; Ward, 2000).

Recommendations

In what follows, we provide recommendations for services and policies that may assist in diminishing the negative impact of EA in Native communities. As social workers, prosecutors, judges, and other professionals are aware, cases of financial exploitation are often difficult to identify and to distinguish in the majority population based on layers of complexity, as well as blurred lines of consent by the elder and intent by the other party (Dessin, 2000). Yet, all professionals serving Native populations or communities are advised to be aware of cultural differences, differentiate between financial exploitation and reciprocal investments by the elders in their family and community, and act in the best interests of Native elders and the communities in which they reside, while being careful not to engage in neocolonialism[5] under the pretext of justice. This is most relevant in the jurisprudence process in which AI/AN communities, families, or individuals are vulnerable to being financially harmed by the very systems in place to protect them, such as when significant resources are extracted from elders, caregivers, and dependent children in multigenerational households through high legal fees and court costs, destabilizing the potentially fragile support and care structures of already vulnerable elders. It is important that jurisprudence and social services systems and processes do no harm as they attempt to help resolve past incidents of EA and prevent future ones.

Most states mandate reporting of suspected EA to APS, and those that do not mandate the reporting strongly urge reporting (NIEJI, 2017). Mandatory reporting for tribes would require that they have the infrastructure in place to which incidents are reported, investigated, and enforced. Currently, very few tribes in non–PL 280 states have the necessary infrastructure to

---

[4] Percentages of children age 19 years and younger by race/ethnicity within their total population as estimated in 2009 are as follows: all races/ethnicities, 27.2%; AI/AN, 33.8%; non-Hispanic Whites, 23.3%; blacks, 32.0%; Asian, 26.1%; Native Hawaiian/Pacific Islander. 33.3%; Hispanic, 37.9%; and two or more races, 50.6% (U.S. Census Bureau, 2012).

[5] Neocolonialism is the process whereby a dominant group exerts indirect control or influence over another group by means of economic and/or political policies rewarding desirable (as defined by the dominant group) behaviors and penalizing undesirable behaviors. For example, policies that are designed to provide financial autonomy or food security to an elder, but that abridge an elder's freedom to contribute resources to help extended family, may be perceived as neocolonialism.

affect mandatory reporting. It is recommended that mandatory reporting through the Indian Health Service and other systems be implemented to ensure assessment and monitoring of potentially harmful circumstances in which older adults reside and to establish a mechanism for data collection to assess the extent of the problem and to be able to evaluate the effects of research-based intervention programs.

SUMMARY

In often tight-knit Native communities, EA is unequivocally a community (rather than simply an individual or dyadic) problem. As this chapter illustrates, this principle holds true in elders' willingness to report (e.g., how will the family be viewed by the community, will the elder or family be harassed, and can the police or justice system handle the matter sufficiently?) as well as responses to abuse (e.g., building closer relationships between vulnerable elders and social services/police, providing education about EA to the community, and using elder councils rather than court systems). Although there is a move toward these traditional, community-focused models, the TLOA creates possibilities for some tribes to work more successfully within the Western legal system, resolving complicated jurisdictional issues that have long prevented the effective arrest and prosecution of perpetrators, as well as providing longer incarcerations to both tribal and nontribal members. Whether various tribes will gravitate more in one direction or the other (traditional or TLOA), or will be able to integrate both, remains to be seen.

REFERENCES

Acierno, R., Hernandez, M. A., Amstadter, A. B., Resnick, H. S., Steve, K., Muzzy, W., & Kilpatrick, D. G. (2010). Prevalence and correlates of emotional, physical, sexual, and financial abuse and potential neglect in the United States: The National Elder Mistreatment Study. *American Journal of Public Health, 100*(2), 292–297. doi:10.2105/AJPH.2009.163089

Acierno, R., Hernandez-Tejado, M. A., Muzzy, W., & Steve, K. (2009). *National Elder Mistreatment Study: Final report*. Washington, DC: U.S. Department of Justice. Retrieved from https://www.ncjrs.gov/pdffiles1/nij/grants/226456.pdf

Allen, S. K., Longhat, M., & Melton, R. (2013). Community policing and social services. Retrieved from https://www.nieji.org/resources/files/operation-golden-shield.pdf

Anisko, B. (2009). Elder abuse in American Indian communities. *American Indian Culture and Research Journal, 33*(3), 43–51. doi:10.17953/aicr.33.3 .b455qt1714213883

Baker, A. (1975). Granny battering. *Modern Geriatric, 8,* 20–24. doi:10.1136/ bmj.3.5983.592-a

Barker, J. C. (2009). Between humans and ghosts. In J. Sokolovsky (Ed.), *The cultural context of aging: Worldwide perspectives* (3rd ed., pp. 606–622). Westport, CT: Praeger.

Beaulaurier, R. L., Seff, L. R., Newman, F. L., & Dunlop, B. (2005). Internal barriers to help seeking for middle-aged and older women who experience intimate partner violence. *Journal of Elder Abuse & Neglect, 17*(3), 53–74. doi:10.1300/J084v17n03_04

Beaulaurier, R. L., Seff, L. R., Newman, F. L., & Dunlop, B. (2007). External barriers to help seeking for older women who experience intimate partner violence. *Journal of Family Violence, 22*(8), 747–755. doi:10.1007/s10896-007-9122-y

Big Foot, D. S., Grant, L., Denton, J., Rhoades, L. P., Sanders, C., CCAN, & USDOJ-OVC. (2000). *Native American elder abuse.* Oklahoma City. PL. Retrieved from http://nicoa.org/wp-content/uploads/2014/05/Native-American -Elder-Abuse-Monograph.pdf

Biolsi, T. (1992). *Organizing the Lakota: The political economy of the New Deal on the Pine Ridge and Rosebud Reservations.* Tucson, AZ: University of Arizona Press.

Brave Heart, M. Y. (2003). The historical trauma response among natives and its relationship with substance abuse: A Lakota illustration. *Journal of Psychoactive Drugs, 35*(1), 7–13. doi:10.1080/02791072.2003.10399988

Brown, A. S. (1989). A survey on elder abuse at one Native American tribe. *Journal of Elder Abuse & Neglect, 1*(2), 17–38. doi:10.1300/J084v01n02_03

Brown, A. S., Fernandez, R. C., & Griffith, T. M. (1990). *Service provider perceptions of elder abuse among the Navajo.* Flagstaff: Northern Arizona University, Social Research Laboratory.

Buchwald, D., Tomita, S., Hartman, S., Furman, R., Dudden, M., & Manson, S. M. (2000). Physical abuse of Urban Native Americans. *Journal of General Internal Medicine, 15,* 562–564. doi:10.1046/j.1525-1497.2000.02359.x

Bureau of Indian Affairs (BIA) & Cloud, L. I. (2016). *Federal register notices: Indian entities recognized and eligible to receive services from the United States Bureau of Indian Affairs.* Washington, DC: Author.

Burston, G. R. (1975). Letter: Granny-battering. *British Medical Journal, 3*(5983), 592. doi:10.1136/bmj.3.5983.592-a

Butler, R. N. (1975). *Why survive? Being old in America.* New York, NY: Harper & Row.

Carson, D. K. (1995). American Indian elder abuse. *Journal of Elder Abuse & Neglect, 7*(1), 17–39. doi:10.1300/J084v07n01_02

Carson, D. K., & Hand, C. (1999). Dilemmas surrounding elder abuse and neglect in Native American communities. In T. Tatara (Ed.), *Understanding elder abuse in minority populations* (pp. 161–186). Philadelphia, PA: Brunner/Mazel.

Cattelino, J. R. (2008). *High stakes: Florida Seminole gaming and sovereignty.* Durham, UK: Duke University Press.

Churchman, C. W. (1967). Guest editorial: Wicked problems. *Management Science, 14*(4), B141–B142. doi:10.1287/mnsc.14.4.B141

Cole, D., & Chaikin, I. (1990). *An iron hand upon the people: The law against the Potlatch on the Northwest Coast.* Vancouver, BC: Douglas & McIntyre, University of Washington Press.

Coon, C. S. (1948). *A reader in general anthropology.* New York, NY: H. Holt.

Cross, J. A. (2014). *A conversation on elder rights.* Paper presented at the 2014 National Title VI Training and Technical Assistance Conference, Washington, DC.

Crowshoe, R., & Manneschmidt, S. (2002). *Akak'stiman: A Blackfoot framework for decision-making and meditation processes* (2nd ed.). Calgary, Alberta, Canada: University of Calgary Press.

Dawes, H. L. (1886). *Senator Dawes's Address.* Washington, DC: Government Printing Office. Retrieved from http://archive.org/stream/annualreport ofbo17unitrich/annualreportofbo17unitrich_djvu.txt

de Jong, M. G., Pieters, R., & Fox, J.-P. (2010). Reducing social desirability bias through item randomized response: An application to measure under-reported desires. *Journal of Marketing Research, 47*(1), 14–27. doi:10.1509/jmkr.47.1.14

Dessin, C. L. (2000). Financial Abuse of the Elderly. *Idaho Law Review, 36*(2), 203–226.

Dumont-Smith, C., & Aboriginal Healing Foundation. (2002). *Aboriginal elder abuse in Canada.* Ottowa, Ontario, Canada: Aboriginal Healing Foundation.

Elliott, E. M. (2011). *Security, with care: Restorative justice and healthy societies.* Halifax, Nova Scotia, Canada: Fernwood Publishing.

Ellis, J. (2009). First nations justice initiatives in Canada. *Totem: The University of Western Ontario Journal of Anthropology, 17*(1), 203–226. Retrieved from https://ir.lib.uwo.ca/totem/vol17/iss1/12

Forer, L. G. (1994). *A rage to punish: The unintended consequences of mandatory sentencing* (1st ed.). New York, NY: W. W. Norton.

Fowler, L. (2004). Politics. In T. Biolsi (Ed.), *Blackwell companions to anthropology: A companion to the anthropology of American Indians* (pp. 69–94). Malden, MA: Blackwell. Retrieved from https://ir.lib.uwo.ca/totem/vol17/iss1/12

Glascock, A. (2009). Is killing necessarily murder? Moral questions surrounding assisted suicide and death. In J. Sokolovsky (Ed.), *The cultural context of aging: Worldwide perspectives* (3rd ed., pp. 77–92). Westport, CT: Praeger.

Gordon, L. (1988). *Heroes of their own lives: The politics and history of family violence: Boston, 1880–1960.* New York, NY: Viking.

Gordon, L. (1994). *Pitied but not entitled: Single mothers and the history of welfare, 1890–1935.* New York, NY: Free Press.

Gray, J. H., & Gregor, W. G. (1878). *China: A history of the laws, manners, and customs of the people.* London, UK: Macmillan.

Hamby, S., Smith, A., Mitchell, K., & Turner, H. (2016). Poly-victimization and resilience portfolios: Trends in violence research that can enhance the understanding and prevention of elder abuse. *Journal of Elder Abuse & Neglect, 28*(4–5), 217–234. doi:10.1080/08946566.2016.1232182

Hand, C. (1996). *Dilemmas Surrounding Elder Abuse and Neglect in Native American Communities.* Paper presented at the 13th Annual Adult Protective Services Conference of the Texas Department of Protective and Regulatory Services and the American Public Welfare Association, San Antonio.

Harmon, A. (2003). American Indians and land monopolies in the Gilded Age. *Journal of American History, 90*(1), 106–133. doi:10.2307/3659793

Haslip, S. (2002). The (re)introduction of restorative justice in Kahnawake: "Beyond indigenization." *Murdoch University Electronic Journal of Law, 9*(1). Retrieved from http://www.murdoch.edu.au/elaw/issues/v9n1/haslip91.html

Heisler, C. J. (2017). Moving forward: Recommendations for advancing late-life polyvictimization practice, policy, and research. *Journal of Elder Abuse & Neglect, 29*(5), 351–363. doi:10.1080/08946566.2017.1388013

Hennessy, C. H., & John, R. (1996). American Indian family caregivers' perceptions of burden and needed support services. *Journal of Applied Gerontology, 15*(3), 275–293. doi:10.1177/073346489601500301

Holkup, P. A., Salois, E. M., Tripp-Reimer, T., & Weinert, C. (2007). Drawing on wisdom from the past: An elder abuse intervention with tribal communities. *Gerontologist, 47*(2), 248–254. doi:10.1093/geront/47.2.248

Hollister, B. A., & Estes, C. L. (2013). Local long-term care Ombudsman Program effectiveness and the measurement of program resources. *Journal of Applied Gerontology, 32*(6), 708–728. doi:10.1177/0733464811434144

Hudson, M. F., Armachain, W. D., Beasley, C. M., & Carlson, J. R. (1998). Elder abuse: Two Native American views. *Gerontologist, 38*(5), 538–548. doi:10.1093/geront/38.5.538

Hudson, M. F., & Carlson, J. R. (1999). Elder abuse: Its meaning to Caucasians, African Americans, and Native Americans. In T. Tatara (Ed.), *Understanding elder abuse in minority populations* (pp. 187–204). Ann Arbor, MI: Taylor & Francis.

Jackson, M. Y., & Sappier, T. (2005). *Elder abuse issues in Indian country.* Washington, DC: Department of Health and Human Services, Administration on Aging.

Jackson, S. L., & Department of Justice. (2016). *Developing an elder abuse case review multidisciplinary team in your community.* Washington, DC: U.S. Department of Justice. Retrieved from https://www.justice.gov/archives/elderjustice/file/938921/download

Jervis, L. L. (2014). Native elder mistreatment. In R. M. T. Rapporteur Institute of Medicine & National Research Council (Eds.), *Elder abuse and its prevention: Forum on global violence prevention, workshop summary* (pp. 75–79). Washington, DC: National Academies Press.

Jervis, L. L., & AI-SUPERPFP Team. (2009). Disillusionment, faith, and cultural traumatization on a Northern Plains reservation. *Traumatology, 15*(1), 11–22. doi:10.1177/1534765608321069

Jervis, L. L., Boland, M. E., & Fickenscher, A. (2010). American Indian family caregivers' experiences with helping elders. *Journal of Cross-Cultural Gerontology, 25*(4), 355–369. doi:10.1007/s10823-010-9131-9

Jervis, L. L., Fickenscher, A., Beals, J., & The Shielding American Indian Elders Project Team. (2014). Assessment of elder mistreatment in two American Indian samples: Psychometric characteristics of the HS-EAST and the native elder life–financial exploitation and –neglect measures. *Journal of Applied Gerontology, 33*(3), 336–356. doi:10.1177/0733464812470748

Jervis, L. L., Sconzert-Hall, W., & Shielding American Indian Elders Project Team. (2017). The conceptualization of mistreatment by older American Indians. *Journal of Elder Abuse & Neglect, 29*(1), 43–58. doi:10.1080/08946566.2016.1249816

Jervis, L. L., Spicer, P., Manson, S. M., & AI-SUPERPFP Team. (2003). Boredom, "trouble," and the realities of postcolonial reservation life. *Ethos, 31*(1), 38–58. doi:10.1525/eth.2003.31.1.38

Knack, M. C. (2004). Women and men. In T. Biolsi (Ed.), *Blackwell companions to anthropology: A companion to the anthropology of American Indians (pp. 51–68).* Malden, MA: Blackwell.

LeResche, D. (1993). Editor's note. *Mediation Quarterly, 10*(4), 321–325. doi:10.1002/crq.3900100402

Litton, L. J., & Ybanez, V. (2015). *Reclaiming what is sacred: Addressing harm to indigenous elders and developing a tribal response to abuse in later life.* Madison, WI: National Clearinghouse on Abuse in Later Life. Retrieved from http://www.ncall.us//FileStream.aspx?FileID=99

Mails, T. E., & Crow, F. (1979). *Fools crow: Wisdom and power.* Tri S Foundation (Ed.). Tulsa, OK: Council Oak Books.

Malley-Morrison, K., & Hines, D. A. (2004). *Family violence in a cultural perspective: Defining, understanding, and combating abuse.* Thousand Oaks, CA: Sage.

Marshall, P. F., & Vaillancourt, M. A. (1993). *Changing the landscape: Ending violence, achieving equality.* Ottowa, Canada: Canadian Panel on Violence Against Women.

Maxwell, E. K., & Maxwell, R. J. (1992). Insults to the body civil: Mistreatment of elderly in two Plains Indian tribes. *Journal of Cross-Cultural Gerontology, 7*(1), 3–23. doi:10.1007/BF00116574

Moore, J. H. (1996). *The Cheyenne.* Cambridge, MA: Blackwell.

Nahmiash, D. (2004). Powerlessness and abuse and neglect of older adults. *Journal of Elder Abuse & Neglect, 14*(1), 21–47. doi:10.1300/J084v14n01_02

National Association of State Units on Aging. (1989, November). *American Indians and elder abuse: Exploring the problem.* Report of a meeting in Albuquerque, NM, convened by the National Aging Resource Center on Elder Abuse. Washington, DC: Author.

National Center on Elder Abuse. (1995, September 24). Addressing elder abuse with American Indian tribes: A national teleconference [Transcript]. Retrieved from https://ncea.acl.gov/resources/docs/archive/Addressing-EA-AI-Tribes-1995.pdf

National Indigenous Elder Justice Initiative (NIEJI). (2017). *Elder abuse codes.* University of North Dakota: Author. Retrieved from http://www.nieji.org/codes

National Institute of Justice. (2007). Indigenous justice systems and tribal society. In *Restorative justice: Perspectives on restorative justice.* Retrieved from http://www.nij.gov/topics/courts/restorative-justice/perspectives/pages/indigenous-tribal.aspx

Nerenberg, L. (1999). Culturally specific outreach in elder abuse. In T. Tatara (Ed.), *Understanding elder abuse in minority populations* (pp. 205–220). Ann Arbor, MI: Taylor & Francis.

Nerenberg, L., Baldridge, D., & Benson, W. F. (2004a). *Elder abuse in Indian country: Research, policy, and practice.* Albuquerque, NM: National Indian Council on Aging. Retrieved from www.nicoa.org/wp-content/uploads/2014/05/elder_abuse_litreview.pdf

Nerenberg, L., Baldridge, D., & Benson, W. F. (2004b). *Preventing and responding to abuse of elders in Indian country.* Albuquerque, NM: National Indian Council on Aging. Retrieved from https://nicoa.org/wp-content/uploads/2016/03/Preventing-and-Responding-to-Abuse-of-Elders-in-Indian-Country.pdf

Oglala Sioux Tribe. (1996 [1984]). Elder abuse code. In *Oglala Sioux Tribe: Law and order code.* Retrieved from http://thorpe.ou.edu/codes/oglala/chapter06-elder.htm

Older Americans Act of 1965, 42 USC 3001, Pub. L. No. 109-365, 218 Stat. Titles I–VII (1965).

Pickering, K. A. (2000). *Lakota culture, world economy.* Lincoln, NE: University of Nebraska Press.

Pillemer, K. (1985). The dangers of dependency: New findings on domestic violence against the elderly. *Social Problems, 33*(2), 146–158. doi:10.2307/800558

Powers, M. N. (1986). *Oglala women: Myth, ritual, and reality.* Chicago, IL: University of Chicago Press.

Prucha, F. P. (1978). *Americanizing the American Indians: Writings by the "friends of the Indian," 1880–1900.* Lincoln, NE: University of Nebraska Press.

Public Law 280, Pub. L. No. ; 28 U.S.C. § 1360; 25 U.S.C. §§ 1321–1326 588–589 (1953).

Ramsey-Klawsnik, H., Heisler, C. J., Gregorie, T., Quinn, K., Roberto, K. A., & Teaster, P. B. (2014). Polyvictimization in later life. *Victimization of the Elderly and Disabled, 17*(1), 3–6. Retrieved from http://www.napsa-now.org/wp-content/uploads/2016/08/701-Polyvictimization-in-Later-Life.pdf

Red Horse, J. G. (1980). Family Structure and Value Orientation in American Indians. *Social Casework: The Journal of Contemporary Social Work, 61*(8), A21–A29. Retrieved from www.dhs.state.mn.us/main/groups/children/documents/pub/dhs16_180056.pdf

Red Horse, J. G. (1983). Indian family values and experiences. In G. J. Powell (Ed.), *The psychosocial development of minority group children* (pp. 258–271). New York, NY: Brunner/Mazel.

Red Horse, J. G. (1997). Traditional American Indian family systems. *Families, Systems, & Health, 15*(3), 243–250. doi:10.1037/h0089828

Rittel, H. W., & Webber, M. M. (1973). Dilemmas in a general theory of planning. *Policy Sciences, 4*(2), 155–169. doi:10.1007/BF01405730

Rittman, M., Kuzmeskus, L. B., & Flum, M. A. (1999). A synthesis of current knowledge on minority elder abuse. In T. Tatara (Ed.), *Understanding elder abuse in minority populations* (pp. 221–238). Philadelphia, PA: Brunner/ Mazel.

Roberto, K. A. (2017). Perpetrators of late life polyvictimization. *Journal of Elder Abuse & Neglect, 29*(5), 313–326. doi:10.1080/08946566.2017.1374223

Salois, E. M., Holkup, P. A., Tripp-Reimer, T., & Weinert, C. (2006). Research as spiritual covenant. *Western Journal of Nursing Research, 28*(5), 505–563. doi:10.1177/0193945906286809

Schweitzer, M. M. (1999). Otoe-missouria grandmothers: Linking past, present, and future. In M. M. Schweitzer (Ed.), *American Indian grandmothers: Traditions and transitions* (1st ed., pp. 159–180). Albuquerque, NM: University of New Mexico Press.

Shipler, L. K., Anand, R., & Hadi, N. (1998). *Cultural considerations in assisting victims of crime: Report on needs and promising practices.* Washington, DC: National MultiCultural Institute.

Smyer, T., & Clark, M. C. (2011). A cultural paradox: Elder abuse in the Native American community. *Home Health Care Management & Practice, 23*(3), 201–206. doi:10.1177/1084822310396971

Sturm, C. (2002). *Blood politics: Race, culture, and identity in the Cherokee nation of Oklahoma.* Berkeley, CA: University of California Press.

Taylor, R. M. (2014). *Elder abuse and its prevention: Workshop summary.* Paper presented at the Forum on Global Violence Prevention, Washington, DC. Retrieved from https://www.nap.edu/catalog/18518/elder-abuse-and-its -prevention-workshop-summary

Teaster, P. B. (2017). A framework for polyvictimization in later life. *Journal of Elder Abuse & Neglect, 29*(5), 289–298. doi:10.1080/08946566.2017.1375444

The National Center on Elder Abuse at The American Public Human Services Association, & Westat Inc. (1998). *The national elder abuse incidence study: Final report.* Washington, DC: U.S. Department of Health and Human Services, Administarion for Children and Families.

Tribal Law and Order Act of 2010, 25 USC, 111th US Congress, HR 725, 124 Stat. 2258 (2010).

Umbreit, M. S. (1989). Crime victims seeking fairness, not revenge: Toward restorative justice. *Federal Probation, 53*(3), 52–57. Retrieved from http:// heinonline.org/HOL/P?h=hein.journals/fedpro53&i=251

U.S. Census Bureau. (2012). Population: Estimates and projections by age, sex, race/ethnicity. Retrieved from https://www.census.gov/compendia/statab/cats/ population/estimates_and_projections_by_age_sex_raceethnicity.html

U.S. Senate Resolution 88-14, United States Senate, 100-981 Sess (1988).

van Ness, D. W. (1990). Restorative justice. In B. Galaway & J. Hudson (Eds.), *Criminal justice, restitution, and reconciliation*. Monsey, NY: Criminal Justice Press.

Wakeling, S., Jorgensen, M., Michaelson, S., & Begay, M. (2001). *Policing on American Indian reservations: A report to the National Institute of Justice*. Washington, DC: U.S. Department of Justice National Criminal Justice Reference Service.

Walsh, C. A., Olson, J. L., Ploeg, J., Lohfeld, L., & MacMillan, H. L. (2010). Elder abuse and oppression: Voices of marginalized elders. *Journal of Elder Abuse & Neglect, 23*(1), 17–42. doi:10.1080/08946566.2011.534705

Ward, D. (2000). Ageism and the abuse of older people in health and social care. *British Journal of Nursing, 9*(9), 560–563. doi:10.12968/bjon.2000.9.9.6292

White, H. B. (2004). Elder abuse in tribal communities. Tucson, AZ: Southwest Center for Law and Policy. Retrieved from http://www.swclap.org/uploads/file/2de3c2e355104a588d680b7e4ad2f4a7/ELDERABUSE.pdf

Wolf, R. V. (2012a). Peacemaking today: Highlights of a roundtable discussion among tribal and state practitioners. Retrieved from http://www.courtinnovation.org/sites/default/files/documents/Peacemaking_Today.pdf

Wolf, R. V. (2012b). Widening the circle: Can peacemaking work outside of tribal communities? Guide for planning. Retrieved from http://www.courtinnovation.org/sites/default/files/documents/PeacemakingPlanning_2012.pdf

Yakima Indian Nation. (1987). *Don't wound my spirit: Yakima Indian Nation's guide to protecting elders from abuse, neglect, and exploitation*. Washington, DC: U. S. Department of Health and Human Services.

6

INTERSECTION OF PUBLIC HEALTH AND NONTRADITIONAL PARTNERS AND APPROACHES TO ADDRESS ELDER ABUSE

Georgia J. Anetzberger

Public health entered the field of elder abuse (EA) after several other systems already had established roots there, giving the problem their own particular approaches and intervention strategies. Public health can assume a leadership role in EA prevention by working with some nontraditional partners and adopting collaborative models familiar to the field.

Chapter Objectives

By the end of this chapter, readers will be able to

1. Understand the potential for public health in EA prevention.

2. Delineate the major approaches to understanding and responding to EA.

3. Describe the role and services of key EA response systems.

4. Illustrate the multidisciplinary imperative as it applies to EA prevention and intervention.

5. Identify current research gaps and practice issues for EA work involving multiple disciplines or systems.

The field of EA can be described as a complex prism. Its many approaches represent the prism sides, each offering a unique perspective on understanding and addressing the problem. EA response systems represent reflections coming from those prism sides, emerging out of the various approaches, with each system assuming specific roles and responsibilities in EA work.

EA as a public health concern is a more recent approach than the others. However, given the increased attention directed toward prevention of EA, the public health system can become an important leader in this field by effectively partnering with nontraditional systems in the process—that is, partnering with systems other than healthcare (its traditional pairing). The intent of this chapter is to identify these nontraditional partners and approaches to EA and to suggest vehicles by which public health can collaborate with them to achieve its EA-related goals.

The chapter begins by discussing seven approaches to EA that have evolved over time, noting their current standing in the field. When considering EA as a public health concern, original research is presented that compares the activities of state public health departments related to EA over a 25-year period. Afterward, the four key EA response systems that represent nontraditional partners to public health are revealed. Their major roles and responsibilities are provided, along with an illustration for how public health might collaborate with each system in fulfilling its EA-related priorities. Possible challenges to these collaborations are given, where appropriate. Then the multidisciplinary imperative to EA is discussed and illustrated through Ohio state and community EA networks and teams wherein public health works cooperatively with nontraditional partners. The chapter ends with suggestions for overcoming barriers to EA work involving multiple disciplines or systems. The existing research gaps in understanding the effectiveness of multidisciplinary EA efforts are included here, too.

Illustrative Case Study

Sally is an only child in her 50s, never married and living alone. She has a career in health services, working two stressful jobs and long hours. It gives her a good income that quickly evaporates with impulse purchases and frequenting of the neighborhood bar. Sally

(continued)

has been in counseling for over a decade. If asked, she responds that her mother drove her to seek help—the woman is so exasperating. Ada is Sally's mother. She is in her late 70s, somewhat frail but living independently in an apartment located a 2-hour drive from Sally. Recently widowed, Ada often is lonely. As a result, she regularly travels by bus to visit Sally, staying in her condominium for a few weeks on each occasion. Time together rarely goes well. Inevitably the two women fight. It usually starts with Ada criticizing Sally for working too hard, spending too freely, and drinking too much. Sally typically reacts with anger and then with a tirade of expletives, accusations, and name-calling. Lately, however, Sally has begun hitting her mother and throwing things at her as well. This has included slapping Ada, punching her, beating her with a stick, throwing books at her, and even pushing her down a short flight of stairs. Injuries have not been serious to date—just a few bruises and a couple of cuts. Still, Ada worries that the situation could get worse. She especially is concerned that Sally could rage and become out of control after one of her evenings at the bar.

ELDER ABUSE APPROACHES AND THEIR HISTORY

The known presence of EA spans centuries, but efforts to understand and respond to it are limited to a few decades. The mistreatment of older adults has been depicted in ethnography, historical record, and literature since preindustrial times (Reinharz, 1986; Stearns, 1986). However, it did not surface as an issue deserving organized intervention in the United States until the 1950s. More surprisingly, EA was the focus of neither scientific nor Congressional inquiry until another quarter century later (Cronin & Allen, 1982; Lau & Kosberg, 1979; U.S. House Select Committee on Aging, 1979). By then it had come to be viewed through many different lenses, resulting in a myriad of distinct approaches, which continue through nowadays.

There are at least seven major approaches to understanding and responding to EA: social problem, medical (geriatric) syndrome, aspect of family (domestic) violence, aging (Aging Network) issue, crime, violation of human rights, and public health concern. The approaches are different from one another in three primary ways: (a) how EA is perceived, (b) which discipline or system has the lead, and (c) which services or programs are most important. The approaches will be described in the order they emerged.

Social Problem

EA was viewed initially as a social problem—that is, a situation seen as incompatible with the values of a significant number of people who are in agreement that collective action is required to alter the situation (Rubington & Weinberg, 1995). During the 1950s and early 1960s a number of urban centers, such as Cleveland and Chicago, became aware of the growing number of older adults, often mentally impaired, who were living alone in the community and outside of institutional settings, without nearby family for support. Concerned about their well-being and fearful that they could suffer self-neglect or exploitation without assistance, social workers led community efforts that eventually resulted in the development of Adult Protective Services (APS) for this population. Modeled after Child Protective Services, APS rests upon social services principles and strategies but recognizes the potential need for legal interventions, particularly those incorporating surrogate decision making, for problem resolution (Anetzberger, 2002).

In the wake of demonstration projects to design and test APS during the late 1960s, the intervention spread nationwide, fueled by the infusion of federal dollars from the 1974 enactment of Title XX of the Social Security Act (Teaster, Wangmo, & Anetzberger, 2010). State legislation followed. Nowadays, there is an APS program in every state. Although the basic structure is the same, there are local variations in such areas as targeted population, reporting requirements, and available funding for services (Anetzberger, 2002). Also, not surprisingly, the first research on EA was conducted by social workers, taking place in one of the urban centers where APS arose—Cleveland. Elizabeth Lau, a protective services supervisor with the county hospital's Chronic Illness Center, and Jordan Kosberg, a member of the social work faculty at Case Western Reserve University, examined cases of older adults seen the past year at the Center and discovered that nearly 10% had experienced EA in some form (Lau & Kosberg, 1979).

Medical Syndrome

Recognition of EA as a geriatric syndrome occurred in spurts beginning in the mid-1970s. The earliest conceptualization can be found in writings published in 1975, describing physical abuse as a "battered old person syndrome" (Butler, 1975) and self-neglect as the "Diogenes syndrome" (Clark, Mankikar, & Gray, 1975). Twenty years later geriatrician Mark Lachs (1995), in an article appearing in the *Journal of Elder Abuse & Neglect*, argued that EA should be regarded as a geriatric syndrome if physicians are to give the issue the level of attention accorded earlier to child abuse. He indicated that, like dementia and depression, EA is characterized as having "several contributing factors that shape patient presentation" rather than one pathophysiologic process (p. 6). Therefore, approaching EA requires definitive diagnosis and management, with interventions geared to the unique combination of impairments that contribute to the patient's presentation, treating what can be improved and recognizing that a cure for the condition may be impossible. Nowadays, physicians such as XinQi Dong, Mark Lachs, and Laura Mosqueda are among the most prominent and prolific researchers in EA. Along with their nursing and other healthcare colleagues, they have advanced the field in such areas as the identification of EA signs and risk factors as well as the development and testing of screening tools and intervention protocols (e.g., Burnes, Pillemer, & Lachs, 2017; Chen & Dong, 2017; Dong, 2015; Mosqueda, Burnight, & Liao, 2005; Rosen et al., 2016; Wiglesworth, Austin, Corona, & Mosqueda, 2009).

Aspect of Family Violence

The first discussions of EA as an aspect of family violence came during the late 1970s. However, recognition that domestic violence programming has an important responsibility for abused elders did not emerge until a decade later. Suzanne Steinmetz (1977), a leading family violence researcher, wrote a section on battered elderly parents in her book *The Cycle of Violence: Assertive, Aggressive and Abusive Family Interaction*. The following year, she presented this population as an overlooked component of family violence in Congressional testimony. Even so, the domestic violence approach did not gain a solid foothold in the EA field until three events converged in the late 1980s and early 1990s. First, Pillemer and Finkelhor (1988) published their groundbreaking metropolitan Boston EA prevalence study, which unexpectedly found spouse abuse to be more than twice as common as abuse by adult children. That same year the Family Violence Prevention and Services Act included older people as potential targets for its program grants. Finally, in 1992, the American Association of Retired Persons' (AARP's) Women's Initiative sponsored a national forum on the concerns of older abused women, bringing together providers from aging services and domestic violence programming. As a result of the forum, AARP funded the Wisconsin Coalition Against Domestic Violence to document the needs of this population and produce a directory of available services, which became a catalyst for promoting recognition and intervention directed at domestic violence in later life.

The domestic violence approach to EA focuses more on abused older women, but does recognize that older men can be abused as well (Kosberg, 2007). It defines the issue as the patterned use of coercive tactics on the part of the perpetrator to gain power and control over the victim. Interventions are aimed at empowering the victim through information, support, and safety planning while working with and holding accountable the perpetrator (Brandl & Raymond, 1997). Nowadays, the National Clearinghouse on Abuse in Later Life serves to galvanize and promote national and local activities directed at older victims of family violence. States and communities vary greatly in creating or adapting domestic violence programs to benefit this population.

Aging Issue

EA as an aging issue suggests that older people are particularly vulnerable to abuse and self-neglect because of conditions or circumstances often associated with later life. These include increased frailty, multiple chronic conditions, loss of social supports, and limited opportunities for income growth.

The perception of EA as an aging issue is best illustrated through the Aging Network, that system of federal, state, and local agencies established by the Older Americans Act (OAA) with the intent of organizing and delivering community-based services for older adults. When enacted in 1965, the OAA had far-reaching objectives but very limited funding and program authorization. Subsequent amendments greatly expanded the functions, services, and reach of the Aging Network, but usually without sufficient accompanying appropriations, especially given the growth of older people as a percentage of the total population (Leadership Council of Aging Organizations, 2011; U.S. General Accounting Office, 1992).

The Aging Network's interest in EA was first articulated in the original legislation's Declaration of Objectives, which include protection against abuse, neglect, and exploitation. Later amendments to the OAA, particularly those passed in 1978, 1987, and 1991, sought to accomplish this objective through programs like the long-term care ombudsman, EA prevention, and national centers on EA and ombudsmen. For those in the Aging Network, EA also reflects the OAA's target populations, where priority is placed on serving those older adults with the greatest social and economic needs (Collins, 1982). Intervention approaches tend to emphasize advocacy for the rights of vulnerable elders, along with public awareness and educational activities and supportive services to prevent EA.

Crime

The "criminalization" of EA began in the late 1980s. Prior to that time, EA primarily was considered a civil, rather than criminal, justice matter when legal interventions were used. However, as other "undesirable" behaviors, such as stalking of women, increasingly came to be regarded as crimes, EA was, too. In this sense, it rode the wave of a larger social trend, moving the issue into the arena of law enforcement, with police and prosecutors taking center stage. Criminalization of EA also came with recognized limitations to the social services approach (Wolf, 2000) and belief that the problem represented "a public concern, not a mere private, family affair" (Heisler, 1991, p. 7).

The intents of the criminal justice approach to EA include maintaining order, protecting society, enforcing law, controlling crime, and punishing perpetrators while still safeguarding their rights (Payne, 2005). In contrast to the other approaches discussed thus far, the focus of criminal justice is minimally on the victim and primarily on the perpetrator. Some states have made EA a crime, whereas in other states prosecution is sought using diverse provisions in the criminal code. The criminal justice approach to EA is evident at the national level through U.S. Department of Justice research, training, and program grants; at the state level through Attorney General Office activities, like Medicaid Fraud Control Units; and in select local communities that have special EA units in prosecutors' offices and dedicated victim advocates.

Violation of Human Rights

Lau and Kosberg's (1979) pioneering research on EA identified violation of rights as one of four forms. However, except for its infliction on residents in care facilities, especially nursing homes, it received little attention until the late 1990s, when EA began to be seen as a global phenomenon. Especially in the new millennium, organizations with broad geographic purpose, such as the United Nations, have become responsive to research showing the problem exists in all world regions. As a result, EA has been embedded in proclamations urging nations to recognize and protect the rights of older people. *Abuse of Older Persons: Recognizing and Responding to Abuse of Older Persons in a Global Context: Report of the Secretary-General* (United Nations, Economic and Social Council, 2002) illustrates this approach. Describing the abuse of older people as a human rights issue, it provides possible responses to the problem. The document was submitted to the Commission for Social Development in preparation for the Second World Assembly on Aging held in Madrid during 2002. The resulting Madrid Plan of Action gives "particular emphasis to the empowerment of older persons, including protection of their rights" (Podnieks, Penhale, Goergen, Biggs, & Han, 2010).

In this approach, EA is seen as an impediment to older adults' ability to defend their basic human and civil rights. Responding to EA requires government action and social will. It usually takes the form of legal statutes and systems for incidence reporting, interventions for preventing the problem and treating its effects, and information centers and hotlines for ensuring that older adults are knowledgeable about their rights (Department of Economic and Social Affairs, 2008).

Public Health Concern

EA as an acknowledged public health concern may have had its origins in a paper presented in 1979 at the 107th Annual Meeting of the American Public Health Association held in New York City. Its authors were two researchers, Tom Hickey and Richard Douglass, the former with his doctorate in public health. The paper revealed findings from their investigation of EA as seen by various professionals providing services to community-dwelling older adults. The research was funded by the Administration on Aging and later published in the association's journal (Hickey & Douglass, 1981). Drs. Hickey and Douglass argued that EA is a serious threat to the public's health. Among their study results, they found that public health professionals (e.g., social workers in health outreach services, public health nurses) were most familiar with such cases. However, subsequent attention by public health did not occur until a decade later at a workshop on family violence convened by U.S. Surgeon General Louis Sullivan. In it, he declared family violence a public health (as well as criminal justice) issue that included the problem of EA (U.S. Office of the Surgeon General, 1986).

A longtime advocate in the field of EA, Nerenberg (2008) is a proponent of the public health approach to EA, describing it in her book *Elder Abuse Prevention: Emerging Trends and Promising Strategies* and citing it as one of five priorities for moving the field forward. Acknowledging public health's emphasis on government as responsible to protect the public, she notes the approach's three prevention strategies: (1) primary (i.e., reducing or eliminating risk factors), (2) secondary (i.e., identifying and treating persons having signs or risk factors for the problem), and (3) tertiary (i.e., stopping the problem, reducing any likely reoccurrence, minimizing its effects, and restoring the functioning of those affected) (Nerenberg, 2008). Typical techniques to accomplish problem prevention include public education, screening, social action, and surveillance.

Research on State Public Health Department Elder Abuse Initiatives

The same year (1989) that Dr. Sullivan declared EA a public health concern, at the urging of a federal public health official, the author helped survey state public health department directors to identify administrative awareness of state EA reporting laws and development of procedures to assist healthcare personnel with their reporting responsibilities (Ehrlich & Anetzberger, 1991). Representatives of all 50 state departments completed the survey or a follow-up telephone interview. The study results revealed that nearly every public health department director ($n = 47$, 94%) was aware of the state EA law. However, just one fifth ($n = 10$, 20%) had written protocols for staff members or community professionals on their reporting obligations. Similarly, only about one quarter ($n = 14$, 28%) of respondents indicated that their departments conducted trainings or awareness campaigns for physicians or nurses on law implementation.

Twenty-five years have passed since this exploratory study, which was first aimed at examining state public health department activities related to EA prevention or intervention. In the meanwhile, the field of EA has progressed, witnessing more and better research to understand the issue along with growth in the number of disciplines and systems having an interest in addressing it. Therefore, it seemed appropriate to conduct another survey of state public health departments to ascertain current involvement in EA work. This time state public health department websites were selected as the target for investigation, because increasingly websites serve to tell the story of the agency represented, describing what it does and identifying partners with which it is linked by virtue of mutual mission or collaborative endeavor.

In January 2014, a systematic survey was undertaken of all 50 state public health department websites plus that of the District of Columbia. This inquiry was confined to answering two questions: (1) Does the website contain information about EA or related interventions, or provide linkage to some other source offering such information? (2) Were any initiatives to address EA identified on the website that involved the state public health department, and if so, were nontraditional partners listed? Survey results were recorded, organized by question, and then checked separately by two investigators, who were particularly attentive to the accuracy, appropriateness, and completeness of items noted.

Survey results revealed that two thirds ($n = 34$, 67%) of state public health department websites included some content on EA. However, in most instances the content was minimal and difficult to access, typically consisting of a link to another agency engaged in EA work that could be found only by using the "right" word in searching the A–Z Index. For example, one state had a link to the EA Protective Services Unit, and another state had a link to a PDF file on long-term care and the Elder Justice Act. Just a handful of state public health department websites ($n = 5$, 10%) offered more extensive information about EA, and the majority of these were states wherein the APS program was housed in the same umbrella department as public health. For instance, one state provided basic information about EA, like forms and signs, along with related linkages. Fewer than one third ($n = 15$, 29%) of state public health department websites mentioned any specific EA initiative in which the department was involved. When something was identified, most often it related to training or education, coalitions, or public awareness. To illustrate, one state listed training in EA prevention, another state noted Local Coordinating Councils on EA, and still another state had a brochure on APS. Nonetheless, rarely was the initiative multidimensional and seldom were partners from other disciplines or systems noted. When they were, those most frequently identified were APS and law enforcement.

Comparing findings from the 1989 study with those from the 2014 study, it seems as if little has changed over a quarter century with respect to the level of attention given EA within state public health departments. State departments seem to recognize the issue, but their activities to prevent it appear quite limited. From a historical perspective, public health may be a relative latecomer to the field of EA. However, its opportunity to elevate the issue and assume a leadership role in EA prevention could not be more timely and important. Moreover, recognition of this vital role has come from several sources, including the Second World Assembly on Aging and the National Policy Summit on Elder Abuse. For instance, the latter's 10 recommendations for federal policy action lead with encouraging the Centers for Disease Control and Prevention (CDC) to recognize EA as a public health issue (National Center on Elder Abuse, 2002). It is important to note that subsequently, and perhaps partly in response to the Summit recommendation, the CDC did recognize EA as a public health issue and publish uniform definitions and recommended data elements (Hall, Karch, Crosby, 2016).

KEY ELDER ABUSE RESPONSE SYSTEMS

The "Elder Abuse Approaches and Their History" section identified several systems active in preventing and intervening in this problem. Healthcare has been a traditional partner and collaborator with public health. The remainder are more likely to represent nontraditional partners or collaborators, at least with respect to EA. This means that public health regularly turns to healthcare, but it less frequently turns to the others. Nontraditional partners have important roles and responsibilities in addressing EA. As such, they can help public health fulfill its EA-related goals and priorities. Moreover, as indicated in the "Multidisciplinary Imperative to Elder Abuse" section later in this chapter, the field of EA has long recognized the importance of disciplines and systems working together for effective action at both case and community levels.

The following subsections briefly describe the key EA response systems and illustrate how public health might benefit from collaborative work with each of them. In addition, possible challenges to this collaboration are noted.

Adult Protective Services

The only response system exclusively concerned with EA (and in most states abuse and neglect of younger adults with disabilities) is APS. Typically operating out of public departments of social services or state units on aging, APS has four primary functions: receive and investigate reports or referrals, evaluate client status (especially endangerment) and service needs, provide or arrange services to prevent or treat harm, and seek legal intervention, if indicated. APS is governed by state law, with variation nationwide. Most such laws mandate reporting by professionals and others in regular contact with older adults, with healthcare providers among those most commonly named. APS primarily embraces the social problem approach to EA. However, depending on political jurisdiction, locally it may assume characteristics of other approaches, particularly as an aging issue and as a crime.

A potential alignment of public health and APS is in the area of EA public education. This key public health technique has been used successfully to discourage such risky behaviors as smoking and drunk driving. It can be applied to help prevent EA by alerting older adults of their potential risk for this problem, identifying examples, and encouraging them to report any occurrence and seek assistance through APS. A possible challenge to collaboration in this arena is found in the typically insufficient funding provided for APS

(Quinn & Benson, 2012) and hence its reluctance at times to increase already strained worker caseloads through the influx of large numbers of new reports arising out of EA awareness campaigns. On the other hand, such campaigns can signal the need for more APS workers and ignite action to address EA.

Domestic Violence and Sexual Assault Programs

Domestic violence and sexual assault programs attempt to ensure the safety of abuse victims and hold perpetrators actionable for their abusive behaviors. Services usually include crisis lines, emergency shelters, transitional housing, legal advocacy, support groups, education, counseling, and information and referral. Most related laws provide criminal penalties for abusers, and civil action to promote the safety and economic security of victims. In this response system EA is seen as an aspect of family violence as well as a crime. Although associated programs are found throughout the country, they tend to be most developed in urban centers, with deficits often found in rural and remote areas.

A likely alignment of public health with domestic violence and sexual assault programs is found in assuring screening for EA as part of annual wellness examinations available to older adults as Medicare recipients, with targeted screening completed more often for such high-risk groups as older adults with dementia and those who are socially isolated. Possible challenges to this collaboration include the relative lack of evidence-based EA interventions and, therefore, the questionable advantage of screening for it. In addition, many domestic violence and sexual assault programs do not address the needs and concerns of older adults, especially the impaired ones. For example, it is not uncommon for shelters to lack handicap accessibility and linkage to aging services.

Aging Network

The Aging Network represents a broad array of supportive, clinical, and life-enhancing services arising out of the OAA. More recently, the Aging Network has focused its attention on long-term services and supports, and added younger adults with disabilities to its service population mix. Structurally, this is reflected in the creation of the Administration for Community Living under the U.S. Department of Health and Human Services, which encompasses the following former separate agencies: Administration on Aging, Office on Disability, and Administration on Developmental

Disabilities. Programmatically, it is illustrated in Aging and Disability Resource Centers, which offer information and assistance to both older people and adults with disabilities in accessing benefits and community services.

Aging Network services include congregate and home-delivered meals, transportation, friendly visiting, socialization, adult day care, personal care, housekeeping, legal services, and the long-term care ombudsman. Assistance for informal caregivers, such as support groups and respite care, is available, too. Many Aging Network services are delivered out of area agencies on aging, county and municipal offices on aging, and senior centers. With respect to EA, Aging Network services can help prevent the problem, providing interventions that address EA risk factors, inhibiting the occurrence or reoccurrence of the problem. In addition, through the long-term care ombudsman, it can address complaints of EA from residents in nursing homes and other residential facilities as well as those from recipients of home and community-based care.

Public health might collaborate with the Aging Network to help inform implementation of evidence-based services and programs, and thereby to improve public policy to prevent EA. The OAA requires the Aging Network to advocate on behalf of services and programs that improve the well-being of older adults and address their needs. It further requires area agencies on aging to have advisory councils to engage in advocacy. Public health also uses social action as a technique to realize its goals. It is a natural alliance for the two systems to come together and advocate in this area of mutual interest and concern. A possible challenge to collaboration at the local level may be found in the lack of established contexts for the two systems to connect regularly and thereby share concerns.

Law Enforcement

Law enforcement addresses violations of the legal code and often is the first responder in crisis situations. It also performs a number of community services, such as well-being checks on impaired older adults. Law enforcement consists of a variety of agencies, including sheriff's departments, municipal police, prosecutor's offices, victim assistance programs, courts, jails, and coroner's offices. For EA, law enforcement may be the first contact in a domestic disturbance or suspicion of severe neglect involving an older adult. It is charged to investigate EA as a crime, and can help APS during its report investigations or use of involuntary interventions, most commonly when the situation is deemed dangerous. Law enforcement has the authority to arrest and prosecute perpetrators as well as to enforce protective or restraining orders. Finally, through victim assistance programs, law enforcement can provide older adult victims of crime with victim compensation information, legal advocacy, counseling, and court accompaniment. This is important because legal options can seem confusing and the justice system daunting without the guidance and assistance of advocates.

Surveillance is a potential area of collaboration between public health and law enforcement. Both systems put much effort into collecting, analyzing, and disseminating data. Therefore, when appropriate it may be beneficial to the field of EA to share and jointly interpret data sets, such as around death reports. Collaboration, however, can be challenging when the definitions used in data collection are incompatible across the two systems and regulations exist to inhibit their alteration.

THE MULTIDISCIPLINARY IMPERATIVE TO ELDER ABUSE

There is widespread agreement that multiple disciplines and systems working in concert with one another are required to effectively address EA (e.g., Dyer, Heisler, Hill, & Kim, 2005; Levi & O'Neill, 1997; Payne, 2002). This perception recognizes the problem's complexity, such as its many definitions, forms, etiologies, and settings. It also acknowledges the various approaches that have evolved to understand EA and the many different systems that respond to it (Anetzberger, 2011). Indeed, the multidisciplinary imperative to EA began more than a half century ago with the development of "protective care" (which eventually would become APS) for older adults and the importance placed from the beginning on social work, medicine, law, and other professions being mutually supportive in helping individuals in need of this type of assistance (O'Neill, 1965; U.S. Department of Health, Education and Welfare, 1961).

The multidisciplinary imperative to EA continues today. At the case level, it primarily takes the form of multidisciplinary (or interdisciplinary) teams (Anetzberger, Dayton, Miller, McGreevey, & Schimer, 2005). Such teams are composed of at least three professionals from different disciplines who come together for clinical case review and recommendation, occasionally also identifying service gaps or system problems. Some teams are generic, considering all EA forms and situations; others are specialized, including those focused on financial abuse or fatality review. At the organizational level, the multidisciplinary imperative is seen in partnerships between agencies (Nerenberg, 1995). Partnerships provide two or more agencies with the ability to formalize their cooperation in areas of mutual interest or concern. Examples of partnerships include interagency agreements and referral protocols. Finally, the multidisciplinary imperative to EA can be seen at the community level in the form of networks (or coalitions). Networks represent the collaborative efforts of many professionals, organizations, and systems to facilitate change in EA prevention or treatment within a municipality, county, region, or state. Networks engage in such activities as public awareness campaigns, professional training and education, program planning, and legislative advocacy (Kasunic & Olson, 2007). They also can be the vehicle for creating and supporting multidisciplinary teams (Teaster et al., 2010).

The multidisciplinary imperative to EA provides public health with an established model and specific options for cooperation with nontraditional partners in achieving EA-related goals and priorities. On the one hand, there are three major benefits to cooperation across disciplines or systems. First, cooperation offers a more holistic perspective for understanding and responding to EA than could be obtained by any single entity. Second, it assures that no discipline or system has sole responsibility for handling the complicated and difficult problem of EA. Third, it forges relations necessary to promote a community-wide approach to EA intervention. On the other hand, working with other disciplines or systems has its challenges, such as potential animosity between their representatives or finding the time required for cooperative endeavors and feeling that the time is well spent.

DISCUSSION BOX

In a time of diminished agency resources with funding cuts and increased service demands with demographic changes, questions often arise about the worth of multidisciplinary efforts. Clearly, EA teams take considerable time and long-term commitment. As such, they compete with team members' work demands and can pose scheduling conflicts. This seems especially true when members must travel significant distances to attend meetings, as often is the case in rural and remote areas, and when there are insufficient other staff available in the agency for task handling when members are away, which often plagues APS and mental health participation. The perceived benefits of multidisciplinary efforts might be greater if there was empirical evidence of their effectiveness. However, such evidence is limited. Forming multidisciplinary teams can be challenging, requiring skilled leadership and dedicated coordination. Maintaining them can prove much more daunting, sometimes resulting in weakened connections among members or even team collapse.

Even so, the benefits of multidisciplinary cooperation are compelling, and tend to outweigh the challenges. These challenges potentially can be overcome with such techniques as the following: remaining focused on the goals of collaboration, accepting needed change, having face-to-face contact, and respecting each other's role and philosophy.

Despite the multidisciplinary imperative's long history and popularity in the field of EA, there is little empirical evidence of its effectiveness. A national survey of EA multidisciplinary teams conducted in the mid-2000s identified none that had been subjected to outcome evaluation (Teaster & Nerenberg, 2004). With one exception, the few subsequent investigations have limited their inquiry to output evaluation and participant satisfaction (e.g., Navarro, Wilber, Yonashiro, & Homeier, 2010; Wiglesworth, Mosqueda, Burnight, Younglove, & Jeske, 2006).

RESEARCH BOX

Twomey et al. discuss the experiences of seven multidisciplinary teams formed in California during the late 2000s through funding from the Archstone Foundation. Although teams were created to meet unique and different needs, they faced similar issues. The authors identify these practical and logistical issues and then present the results of an output evaluation conducted across teams. Illustration of such issues follows:

- Membership: Should team membership be open or restricted?

- Leadership: What qualities are important in the person who plays the key role in establishing the team?

- Sponsorship: What are the essential characteristics of the team's host agency?

- Coordinator: What is the team coordinator's role?

- Confidentiality: How can the team keep confidential the personal information of clients discussed during case consultation?

- Data collection: What data should be gathered?

Overall, the seven teams demonstrated notable productivity during their first 2 years of operations. For example, together they held more than 1,000 infrastructure development meetings, trained

---

(continued)

5,575 individuals, recruited 109 volunteers, conducted 957 assessments or screenings, and participated in 103 media events. The authors conclude by speculating about the future for EA multidisciplinary teams, such as their ability to consult on complex ethical matters and how new technologies may enhance team operations.

The notable exception is a rigorous outcome evaluation of the effectiveness of a multidisciplinary EA forensic center for holding financial abusers accountable through referral for criminal prosecution. The results suggest that victim situations examined by the forensic center were 10 times more likely than a matched population receiving usual care from APS to be referred to the local district attorney's office for case review and ultimate filing and conviction (Navarro, Gassoumis, & Wilber, 2013).

OHIO EXAMPLES OF THE MULTIDISCIPLINARY IMPERATIVE TO ELDER ABUSE

Ohio was among the first states to use a multidisciplinary approach to address EA. Work of this nature began in the 1960s when the Welfare Federation (now called the Center for Community Solutions) convened local agency directors in Cleveland to develop protective care for vulnerable older adults. This same organization eventually led in establishing the nation's oldest multidisciplinary community and state coalitions, the Consortium Against Adult Abuse (formed in 1980; www.c3a5county.org) and Ohio Coalition for APS (formed in 1984; www.ocapsohio.org), respectively. For this reason, Ohio provides useful illustrations of the multidisciplinary imperative to address EA and how public health has worked with nontraditional partners to respond to this problem. Both state and community initiatives are described as follows.

There are two EA multidisciplinary efforts at the state level with public health involvement. The first is the Ohio Attorney General's Elder Abuse Commission. The Commission was established in 2009, building on the previous work of the Ohio Elder Abuse Policy Summit, which resulted in the formation of the Ohio Attorney General's Elder Abuse Task Force. Its purpose is to improve education, boost research, and raise awareness about EA in the state. Comprising representatives from 14 state government agencies (including the Ohio Department of Health) and 16 stakeholder organizations (such as AARP), the Commission meets quarterly, with committees convened more often as needed. Commission activities have included a statewide forum to promote more and better EA research as well as legislation to update and expand the state's APS law. In the latter regard, the proposed policy would add several new categories of mandatory reporters, including employees of health departments operated by city boards of health or general health districts.

The second state-level multidisciplinary initiative concerned with EA is the Ohio Family Violence Prevention Project. First formed in 2007 with funding from the Anthem Foundation of Ohio (now called the Health-Path Foundation), the Project was led by the Ohio State University School of Public Health and the Health Policy Institute of Ohio. It actively involved a Working Group comprising state agency officials, local practitioners, and researchers, including representation from the Ohio Department of Health. The Project's goal was to increase awareness of family violence among government leaders and agency officials, thereby building support for family violence prevention. Activities to accomplish this goal focused on identifying, accessing, analyzing, and summarizing existing data sets on child abuse, intimate partner violence, and EA, with application for the state as a whole as well as individual regions and counties. The resulting products were widely disseminated. They included County Profiles, a State Surveillance Report with recommendations for improving family violence prevention in Ohio (Health Policy Institute of Ohio, 2008), and County Report Cards given out at regional workshops aimed at training local family violence professionals on how to use the data. The most recent iteration of the Project began in February 2014 and planned to cover a 14-month period. The funder, goal, key personnel, representative organizations, and most activities were the same as in 2007. This time, however, the emphasis was on updating the data, expanding the problem to include bullying, and institutionalizing the effort to ensure its continuance in the future.

Two community-level multidisciplinary efforts to influence EA case assessment and service delivery are found in Cuyahoga County or greater Cleveland. Both recognize the importance of public health involvement and include representatives of public health as members. The first is the Hoarding Connection of Cuyahoga County (www.hoardingconnectioncc.org), with the County Board of Health identified as one of three organizing partners (Anetzberger, 2017). Compulsive hoarding severity increases with each decade of life, with self-neglect common among elderly hoarders (Ayers, Saxena, Golshan, & Wetherell, 2010; Dong, Simon, Mosqueda, & Evans, 2012). Self-neglect and self-abuse are under the umbrella of EA, along with elder mistreatment by trusted others and fraud and scams by strangers and acquaintances (Anetzberger, 2012). The Hoarding Connection's mission is to educate the community about the need for a coordinated effort of personnel from local government, mental health, and social services agencies to effectively help individuals who hoard and those working with them. It has 24 partnering agencies that come together and use the Enforced Harm Reduction model for long-term management of local hoarding situations. This model relies on an interdisciplinary team of housing enforcement and services providers working with the person who hoards. The intent of intervention is to reach a level of safety and well-being that is absent when living with too much stuff, in the process benefiting the community by removing hazards and improving property values. The Hoarding Connection has an annual conference to which multiple disciplines and systems are invited.

The second community-level multidisciplinary example is the Cuyahoga County APS Interdisciplinary Team (I Team), with public hospital, health, and mental health members on its steering committee and case consultation team. The I Team was launched in 2011 in the wake of efforts by the Ohio Supreme Court's Subcommittee on Adult Guardianship to establish such teams in each of the state's 88 counties. Currently more than half have them.

POLICY BOX

Ohio has considered enacting legislation that would mandate the creation of local I teams to improve community response to EA victims. Such legislation originally was recommended in the mid-2000s in the state Attorney General's Elder Abuse Task Force Report (Ohio Attorney General, 2005) and subsequently introduced in sessions of the Ohio General Assembly, but initially not enacted. As conceived, I teams would address issues that cross systems. They would be bound through a memorandum of understanding signed by all members. Modeled after Wisconsin's experience (described in the Report), Ohio local I teams would comprise a group of professionals from varied disciplines who meet regularly to discuss and provide consultation on specific cases of EA. I team members collectively would determine the best service plan for each case, recognizing that the remedy for the problem transcends disciplines

---

(continued)

<u>POLICY BOX</u> (*continued*)

and requires joint effort. As noted elsewhere in this chapter, like Wisconsin, Kentucky mandates the use of I teams. Many Ohio advocates believe that it is only through law passage that interdisciplinary action will be assured and the processes for collaborative case response maintained. In 2015, Ohio enacted a law mandating that each county forms an APS I Team, a decade after initial introduction of such legislation; it was a long-fought victory for Ohio advocates of the multidisciplinary model for addressing EA.

Cuyahoga County's I TEAM represents a joint endeavor of the local APS program and county probate court. Its goal is to create a collaboration that will improve each lead EA agency's response to victims of abuse, neglect, and exploitation. More specifically, the I Team reviews cases where prior interventions proved unsuccessful, promotes communication and coordination between agencies, seeks to enhance the knowledge and skills of its members, and identifies system problems and possible solutions. The I Team has 57 members, representing all key EA response systems plus others such as higher education, veterans' services, and programming for persons with developmental disabilities.

A recent evaluation of the I Team suggests that members are highly satisfied with its composition, structure, and functioning. However, they indicate a need for improvement in all areas of potential impact. One fourth of respondents feel that there are unmet needs or areas for improvement in relation to public policy/agency issues, communication/collaboration, and knowledge. Nearly one half see deficits in client outcomes. In particular, they want the I Team to improve its ability to prevent EA and to shorten the time required for clients to receive services (Margaret Blenkner Research Institute, 2013).

THE FUTURE OF MULTIDISCIPLINARY COLLABORATION TO ADDRESS ELDER ABUSE

Multidisciplinary collaboration is believed to be essential for understanding and addressing all complex problems, including EA. Sometimes, it is seen to be even more important in this field than other aspects of family violence or even most health issues because of the many, and growing, number of approaches, systems, disciplines, and laws that relate to EA. The multidisciplinary imperative is further underscored by the lack of sound empirical research that shows the effectiveness of any particular intervention. Even with such evidence, it is improbable that other systems or laws would give way to the one showing better outcomes. Therefore, the current situation is likely to remain. This means that disciplines and systems will have to learn to work together, identifying the contexts and processes that provide the most efficient operations and desired results for EA victims.

What currently exists to guide multidisciplinary collaboration in EA are various sets of recommended strategies from those who have experienced or observed such networks, interagency agreements, or teams. Next is a sample of recommendations spanning three decades. In many regards, they offer a similar message—belief in collective action and recognition that each member plays a valuable role in the realization of group goals.

- Bernotavicz (1982) emphasizes having a common purpose and goals, competent leadership, strong belief in the worth of collaboration, solid infrastructure, valuing the contribution of others, mutual accountability, open communication, and a results-oriented approach.

- Dayton, Anetzberger, and Matthey (1997) suggest focusing on positive experiences, resolving problems early, seeking and accepting help when needed, recognizing the interdependency of disciplines and organizations, opening up to other agencies, never criticizing other professionals or organizations, believing that the best planning and problem solving is done collectively, and starting with small projects that have a high likelihood of success.

- Koenig, Leiste, Spano, and Chapin (2013) stress the importance of how team members work together to address issues like role conflict, agency policies that define team members' involvement, external support, and the capacity of individual team members to develop trust with older adults receiving team services.

Literature review suggests that empirical evidence that shows what works and what does not work in EA prevention and intervention is lacking

(Ploeg, Fear, Hutchison, MacMillan, & Bolan, 2009). The recent addition of a single study discussed earlier in this chapter that demonstrates desired outcomes through a forensic center does little to prove the worth of multidisciplinary interventions overall. As recommended by Dong (2012, p. 39), "more systematic studies are needed" on multidisciplinary teams, particularly rigorously designed investigations that consider measures of relevant outcomes. Certainly, there are many research questions that need answers to justify or refine the use of such collaborations, including which team composition is most effective for which desired outcome and whether having paid professional staff actually promotes more positive results than the lack of it. As EA recognition continues to grow and reports of this problem's occurrence increase, finding answers to fundamental questions about interventions becomes more and more critical.

SUMMARY

There are seven major approaches for understanding and responding to EA. Beginning with the view that EA is a social problem through its perception as a public health concern, these varied approaches have resulted in different professional disciplines and systems putting their particular "mark" on how to best address EA. Public health is a more recent system to assume a leadership role in this field. As such, it must work with some nontraditional partners, such as APS and law enforcement, if it expects to fulfill its EA-related priorities. Working together means recognizing the roles and responsibilities of these partners and identifying potential alignments for collaboration. These reflect some of public health's core functions. In this light, the long-standing multidisciplinary imperative to EA intervention provides a model for public health to use in working across disciplines and systems. In EA the multidisciplinary model most commonly assumes the form of community networks, interagency agreements, and case consultation teams, as illustrated in select Ohio initiatives. The field of EA would benefit from more development and rigorous evaluation of interventions to learn what works and what does not work in preventing this problem. Therefore, it is not surprising that little research exists to support this model. However, in a field crowded with distinct approaches and systems, the multidisciplinary model represents a promising practice for EA prevention and intervention, and the one most likely to prevail.

Thought-Provoking Questions

1. What activities could the department of health in your state undertake to increase awareness about EA? Which state agencies should the department select as partners in these activities?

2. What has your county or municipality done to promote or improve collaboration across agencies on behalf of EA victims? What more should be done?

3. If you were asked to organize a multidisciplinary EA case consultation team, which professional disciplines would you include? Would any of them be challenging to find or engage?

4. What data sets are available to estimate the prevalence and incidence of EA locally? What more are required to indicate the scope of this problem?

5. Sometimes new laws and policies are necessary to address problems. Are any needed in your state to improve the identification, prevention, or treatment of EA?

REFERENCES

Anetzberger, G. J. (2002). Adult protective services. In D. J. Ekerdt (Ed.), *The Macmillan encyclopedia of aging* (pp. 14–17). New York, NY: Macmillan.

Anetzberger, G. J. (2011). The evolution of a multidisciplinary response to elder abuse. *Marquette Elder's Advisor, 13*(1), 107–128.

Anetzberger, G. J. (2012). An update on the nature and scope of elder abuse. *Generations, 36*(3), 12–20.

Anetzberger, G. J. (2017). Elder abuse multidisciplinary teams. In X. Dong (Ed.), *Elder abuse: Research, practice and policy* (pp. 417–432). Cham, Switzerland: Springer International Publishing.

Anetzberger, G. J., Dayton, C., Miller, C. A., McGreevey, J. F., Jr., & Schimer, M. (2005). Multidisciplinary teams in the clinical management of elder abuse. *Clinical Gerontologist, 28*(1/2), 157–171. doi:10.1300/J018v28n01_08

Ayers, C. R., Saxena, S., Golshan, S., & Wetherell, J. L. (2010). Age at onset and clinical features of late life compulsive hoarding. *International Journal of Geriatric Psychiatry, 25*(2), 142–149. doi:10.1002/gps.2310

Bernotavicz, F. (1982). Community role. In *Improving protective services for older Americans: A national guide series*. Portland: University of Southern Maine.

Brandl, B., & Raymond, J. (1997). Unrecognized elder abuse victims: Older abused women. *Journal of Case Management, 6*(2), 62–68.

Burnes, D., Pillemer, K., & Lachs, M. S. (2017). Elder abuse severity: A critical but understudied dimension of victimization for clinicians and researchers. *Gerontologist, 57*(4), 745–756. doi:10.1093/geront/gnv688

Butler, R. N. (1975). *Why survive? Being old in America.* New York, NY: Harper & Row.

Chen, R., & Dong, X. (2017). Risk factors of elder abuse. In X. Dong (Ed.), *Elder abuse: Research, practice and policy* (pp. 93–107). Cham, Switzerland: Springer International Publishing.

Clark, A. N. G., Mankikar, G. D, & Gray, I. (1975). Diogenes syndrome: A clinical study of gross neglect in old age. *Lancet, 1*(7903), 366–368.

Collins, M. (1982). Aging network role. In *Improving protective services for older Americans: A national guide series.* Portland, ME: University of Southern Maine.

Cronin, R., & Allen, B. (1982). *The uses of research sponsored by the Administration on Aging (AoA): Maltreatment and abuse of the elderly* (Case Study no. 5). Washington, DC: Gerontological Research Institute.

Dayton, C., Anetzberger, G. J., & Matthey, D. (1997). A model for service coordination between mental health and adult protective services. *Journal of Mental Health and Aging, 3*(3), 295–308.

Department of Economic and Social Affairs. (2008). *Guide to the national implementation of the Madrid International Plan of Action on Ageing.* New York, NY: United Nations.

Dong, X. (2012). Future directions for elder abuse: Advancing research, education, and training, and continued policy efforts. *Public Policy & Aging Report, 22*(1), 37–41. doi:10.1093/ppar/22.1.37

Dong, X. (2015). Elder abuse: Systematic review and implications for practice. *Journal of the American Geriatrics Society, 63,* 1214–1238. doi:10.1111/jgs.13454

Dong, X., Simon, M. A., Mosqueda, L., & Evans, D. A. (2012). The prevalence of elder self-neglect in a community-dwelling population: Hoarding, hygiene, and environmental hazards. *Journal of Aging and Health, 24*(3), 507–524. doi:10.1177/0898264311425597

Dyer, C. B., Heisler, C. J., Hill, C. A., & Kim, L. C. (2005). Community approaches to elder abuse. *Clinics in Geriatric Medicine, 21*(2), 429–447. doi:10.1016/j.cger.2004.10.007

Ehrlich, P., & Anetzberger, G. (1991). Survey of state public health departments on procedures for reporting elder abuse. *Public Health Reports, 106*(2), 151–154. Retrieved from https://www.ncbi.nlm.nih.gov/pmc/articles/PMC1580213

Hall, J. E., Karch, D. L., & Crosby, A. E. (2016). *Elder abuse surveillance: Uniform definitions and recommended core data elements, version 1.0.* Atlanta, GA: Centers for Disease Control and Prevention.

Health Policy Institute of Ohio. (2008). *White paper on improving family violence prevention in Ohio.* Columbus: Author.

Heisler, C. J. (1991). The role of the criminal justice system in elder abuse cases. *Journal of Elder Abuse & Neglect, 3*(1), 5–33. doi:10.1300/J084v03n01_02

Hickey, T., & Douglass, R. L. (1981). Mistreatment of the elderly in the domestic setting: An exploratory study. *American Journal of Public Health, 71*, 500–507. doi:10.2105/AJPH.71.5.500

Kasunic, M. L., & Olson, T. (2007). *National Committee for the Prevention of Elder Abuse elder abuse prevention local network development project 2004–2007: Final report years 1–3.* Phoenix, AZ: Area Agency on Aging Region One.

Koenig, T. L., Leiste, M. R., Spano, R., & Chapin, R. K. (2013). Multidisciplinary team perspectives on older adult hoarding and mental illness. *Journal of Elder Abuse & Neglect, 25*, 56–75. doi:10.1080/08946566.2012.712856

Kosberg, J. I. (Ed.). (2007). *Abuse of older men.* Binghamton, NY: Haworth Maltreatment & Trauma Press.

Lachs, M. S. (1995). Preaching to the unconverted: Educating physicians about elder abuse. *Journal of Elder Abuse & Neglect, 7*(4), 1–12. doi:10.1300/J084v07n04_01

Lau, E. E., & Kosberg, J. I. (1979). Abuse of the elderly by informal care providers. *Aging, 299*, 10–15.

Leadership Council of Aging Organizations. (2011). Consensus recommendations for the 2011 Older Americans Act reauthorization. Retrieved from www .LCAO.org

Levitt, S., & O'Neill, R. (1997). A call for a functional multidisciplinary approach to intervention in cases of elder abuse, neglect, and exploitation: One legal clinic's experience. *Elder Law Journal, 5*(1), 195–212.

Margaret Blenkner Research Institute. (2013). *Evaluation of the Cuyahoga County Adult Protective Services Interdisciplinary Team: Final report.* Cleveland, OH: Benjamin Rose Institute on Aging.

Mosqueda, L., Burnight, K., & Liao, K. (2005). The life cycle of bruises in older adults. *Journal of the American Geriatrics Society, 53*, 1339–1343. doi:10.1111/j.1532-5415.2005.53406.x

National Center of Elder Abuse. (2002). *National Policy Summit on Elder Abuse: Proceedings.* Washington, DC: National Association of State Units on Aging.

Navarro, A. E., Gassoumis, Z. D., & Wilber, K. H. (2013). Holding abusers accountable: An elder abuse forensic center increases criminal prosecution of financial exploitation. *Gerontologist, 53*(2), 303–312. doi:10.1093/geront/gns075

Navarro, A. E., Wilber, K. H., Yonashiro, J., & Homeier, D. C. (2010). Do we really need another meeting? Lessons from the Los Angeles County Elder Abuse Forensic Center. *Gerontologist, 50*(5), 702–711. doi:10.1093/geront/gnq018

Nerenberg, L. (1995). *Building partnerships: A guide to developing coalitions, interagency agreements and teams in the field of elder abuse.* Washington, DC: National Center on Elder Abuse.

Nerenberg, L. (2008). *Elder abuse prevention: Emerging trends and promising strategies.* New York, NY: Springer Publishing.

Ohio Attorney General. (2005). *Ohio Elder Abuse Task Force report*. Columbus: Author.

O'Neill, V. (1965). Protecting older people. *Public Welfare, 23*(2), 119–127.

Payne, B. K. (2002). An integrated understanding of elder abuse and neglect. *Journal of Criminal Justice, 30*, 535–547. doi:10.1016/S0047-2352(02)00175-7

Payne, B. K. (2005). *Crime and elder abuse: An integrated perspective* (2nd ed.). Springfield, IL: Charles C. Thomas Publisher. doi:10.1080/00981380801970368

Pillemer, K., & Finkelhor, D. (1988). The prevalence of elder abuse: A random sample survey. *Gerontologist, 28*(1), 51–57. doi:10.1093/geront/28.1.51

Ploeg, J., Fear, J., Hutchison, B., MacMillan, H., & Bolan, G. (2009). A systematic review of interventions for elder abuse. *Journal of Elder Abuse & Neglect, 21*, 187–210. doi:10.1080/08946560902997181

Podnieks, E., Penhale, B., Goergen, T., Biggs, S., & Han, D. (2010). Elder mistreatment: An international narrative. *Journal of Elder Abuse & Neglect, 22*, 131–163. doi:10.1080/08946560903436403

Quinn, K. M., & Benson, W. F. (2012). The states' elder abuse victim services: A system still in search of support. *Generations, 36*(3), 66–72.

Reinharz, S. (1986). Loving and hating one's elders: Twin themes in legend and literature. In K. A. Pillemer & R. S. Wolf (Eds.), *Elder abuse: Conflict in the family* (pp. 25–48). Dover, MA: Auburn House.

Rosen, T., Lachs, M. S., Teresi, J., Eimicke, J., Van Haitsma, K., & Pillemer, K. (2016). Staff-reported strategies for prevention and management of resident-to-resident elder mistreatment in long-term care facilities. *Journal of Elder Abuse & Neglect, 28*(1), 1–13. doi:10.1080/08946566.2015.1029659

Rubington, E., & Weinberg, M. S. (Eds.). (1995). *The study of social problems: Seven perspectives* (5th ed.). New York, NY: Oxford University Press.

Stearns, P. J. (1986). Old age family conflict: The perspective of the past. In K. A. Pillemer & R. S. Wolf (Eds.), *Elder abuse: Conflict in the family* (pp. 3–24). Dover, MA: Auburn House.

Steinmetz, S. K. (1977). *The cycle of violence: Assertive, aggressive, and abusive family interaction*. New York, NY: Praeger.

Teaster, P. B., & Nerenberg, L. (2004). *A national look at elder abuse multidisciplinary teams*. Washington, DC: National Committee for the Prevention of Elder Abuse.

Teaster, P. B., Wangmo, T., & Anetzberger, G. J. (2010). A glass half full: The dubious history of elder abuse policy. *Journal of Elder Abuse & Neglect, 22*(1-2), 6–15. doi:10.1080/08946560903436130

Twomey, M. S., Jackson, G., Li, H., Marino, T., Melchior, L. A., Randolph, J. F., . . . Wysong, J. (2010). The successes and challenges of seven multidisciplinary teams. *Journal of Elder Abuse & Neglect, 22*, 291–305. doi:10.1080/08946566 .2010.490144

United Nations, Economic and Social Council. (2002). *Abuse of older persons: Recognizing and responding to abuse of older persons in a global context: Report of the Secretary-General*. New York, NY: United Nations.

U.S. Department of Health, Education and Welfare. (1961). *The nation and its older people: Report of the White House Conference on Aging.* Washington, DC: Government Printing Office.

U.S. General Accounting Office. (1992). *Administration on Aging: Harmonizing growing demands and shrinking resources* (GAO/PEMD-92-7). Gaithersburg, MD: Author.

U.S. House Select Committee on Aging. (1979). *Elder abuse: The hidden problem* (Comm. Pub. No. 96-220). Washington, DC: Government Printing Office.

U.S. Office of the Surgeon General. (1986). *Report: Surgeon General's workshop on violence and public health.* Washington, DC: U.S. Health Resources and Services Administration.

Wiglesworth, A., Austin, R., Corona, M., & Mosqueda, L. (2009). *Bruising as a forensic marker of physical elder abuse.* Washington, DC: U.S. Department of Justice.

Wiglesworth, A., Mosqueda, L., Burnight, K., Younglove, T., & Jeske, D. (2006). Findings from an elder abuse forensic center. *Gerontologist, 46*(2), 277–283. doi:10.1093/geront/46.2.277

Wolf, R. S. (2000). Elders as victims of crime, abuse, neglect, and exploitation. In M. B. Rothman, B. D. Dunlop, & P. Entzel (Eds.), *Elders, crime, and the criminal justice system: Myth, perceptions, and reality in the 21st century* (pp. 19–42). New York, NY: Springer Publishing.

7

INITIATIVES, ORGANIZATIONS, AND EFFORTS ADDRESSING ELDER ABUSE

Pamela B. Teaster, Jeffrey E. Hall, and Fatemeh Zarghami

Chapter Objectives

By the end of this chapter, readers will be able to

1. Describe key agencies and organizations addressing elder abuse.

2. Explain the influence of nationally visible cases of elder abuse.

3. Understand the usefulness of resources related to elder abuse.

With assistance of federal and nonfederal agencies and entities, the issue of elder abuse (EA) is capturing more and more public attention. However, the efforts to keep the problem visible will continue to be waged by effectively demonstrating and communicating that the problem can be successfully addressed. This chapter provides information about major federal initiatives and resources related to EA, the work of important national organizations advancing EA prevention, and relevant efforts conducted at the individual level. The chapter concludes with suggestions for future directions for attention.

Disclaimer: The findings and conclusions in this chapter are those of the authors and do not necessarily represent the official position of the Centers for Disease Control and Prevention.

In 2000, Rosalie Wolf (p. 6), founding mother of the EA movement, opined:

Almost a quarter century has passed since elder abuse first became a matter of public concern. Although the topic had surfaced briefly in British medical journals in the mid-1970s, testimony about "parent battering" at a U.S. congressional subcommittee hearing on family violence in 1978 (U.S. House of Representatives, 1978) brought elder abuse from behind closed doors onto the national stage. Once elder abuse was linked to family violence, it became a hot topic in the media.

More than a decade later, Anetzberger (2012) wrote a follow-up article in which she discussed research advancements in the field. She observed that, although much progress had been made, "It may be difficult to refine the definition of elder abuse because of existing prevention and detection programs, but studies are under way that will affect our understanding of this complex problem" (p. 12). In recognition of this complexity and the need to elevate the status of the problem of EA, practitioners and academics began to stress that EA should be recognized as a public health issue. The earliest formal, coordinated effort to achieve this recognition occurred during the convention of the first National Summit on Elder Abuse in 2001.

In light of this imprimatur, which is now decades old, this chapter highlights organizations and initiatives related to EA, which provide persons working in public health with an orientation to important actions taken to address this problem. We specifically describe functions performed by an array of prominent programs that attempt to prevent EA. The information presented in this chapter will allow the reader to develop an understanding of efforts by selected organizations that wish to protect the well-being of older adults; to understand the unique features of initiatives and actions; and to elucidate areas of possible synergy with existing or planned public health strategies, programs, or initiatives. This understanding could, in turn, stimulate innovative thought about the ways that public health might add to, build upon, or enhance these efforts. For our purposes, this chapter includes components of activities and initiatives intended to do the following:

- Raise awareness and educate about different methods to prevent EA

- Develop knowledge, skills, and abilities to promote EA prevention

- Encourage development of professional careers with focus on promotion of older adults' health

- Create robust, sustainable systems, organizational arrangements, infrastructures, or environments within relevant sectors and settings

- Support and enhance effective efforts to

  - Decrease the likelihood of EA among high-risk adults by reducing perpetration and addressing age or health-related vulnerabilities

  - Detect and investigate other potential cases of EA

  - Optimize favorable and positive outcomes when addressing substantiated EA cases

The initiatives, organizations, and efforts discussed in this chapter are by no means inclusive of all entities and activities addressing EA. Rather, we provide examples of noteworthy organizations and endeavors with discernable linkages to tenets of public health and with which the chapter authors are familiar. We selected the following major federal initiatives for inclusion: Administration on Aging (AoA)/Administration for Community Living (ACL), Centers for Disease Control and Prevention (CDC), Centers for Medicare and Medicaid Services (CMS), Department of Justice (DOJ), and Substance Abuse and Mental Health Services Administration (SAMHSA). Next, we discuss national organizations specifically concerned with EA (i.e., AARP, National Committee for the Prevention of Elder Abuse [NCPEA], International Committee for the Prevention of Elder Abuse, National Adult Protective Services Association [NAPSA]), followed by some other national organizations addressing the EA problem (i.e., American Bar Association [ABA] Committee on Law and Aging, National Clearinghouse on Abuse in Later Life [NCALL], and International Network for the Prevention of Elder Abuse [INPEA]). Using the same selection criteria, we then describe initiatives: Safe Havens, World Day on EA, and awareness raising by celebrities. The chapter concludes with suggestions for future directions for campaigns and model programs in the coming years.

NATIONAL ENTITIES AND INITIATIVES WITH PUBLIC HEALTH INTERSECTIONS

Nascent efforts addressing EA are associated with Public Welfare Amendments to the Social Security Act (SSA, 1962) authorizing payments to states to establish protective services for persons "with physical and/or mental limitations, who were unable to manage their own affairs or who were neglected or exploited." According to Blenkner, Bloom, and Nielses (1972), those who received protective services had a higher mortality rate and higher nursing home placement rate than those who received traditional services, which suggested that enriched, protective services actually worsened client outcomes rather than improved them. Advocates for the system continued their work in the Congress, despite the findings of the Blenkner et al. study, the similar conclusions of its subsequent reanalysis by Berger and Piliavin (1976), and the existence of earlier findings showing protective services units to be costly and of questionable effect (U.S. Department of Health, Education, and Welfare, 1966). Congress amended the SSA in 1974 regarding the mandated protective service units in all states for adults aged 18 years and older (Wolf, 2003).

The aforementioned, counterintuitive results were not convincing enough proof that older and vulnerable persons would not benefit from state protection and intervention. Consequently, over time, APS programs were developed in each state and became inextricably linked to EA. Because APS is composed predominantly of social workers, this important linkage spurred a recognition of EA as a social problem (see Chapter 6). Over time, the understanding of EA became broader, and the topic expanded well beyond its disciplinary genesis to involve the fields of medicine, law, gerontology, and public health, along with many other subfields that continue to expand to the present day, as evidenced by the proliferation of federal programs addressing the matter. In this context, EA shifted from being conceived as a problem with solely social implications to one with clear implications for the health and well-being of the entire populace. Next, we present selected initiatives enacted by federal agencies.

Administration for Community Living

The Administration for Community Living (ACL; earlier known as the Administration on Aging or AoA) includes a number of programs that address EA. One of these is NCEA, a resource for policy makers, social services and healthcare practitioners, the justice system, researchers, advocates, and families. The NCEA is directed by the U.S. Administration for Community Living. Another program is the Office of Elder Justice and Adult Protective Services. This office manages the operation, administration, and assessment of EA prevention, legal assistance development, and pension counseling programs funded through the Older Americans Act (OAA). The office also leads the development and implementation of comprehensive APS systems to provide a coordinated and seamless response for helping adult victims of abuse and preventing abuse before it happens.

Clearinghouse on Abuse and Neglect of the Elderly (CANE). From 1988 to 2010, AoA/ACL provided funding to the University of Delaware to establish and maintain CANE. Fully computerized, CANE is the nation's largest archive of published research, training resources, government documents, and other sources on EA. With more than 5,000 holdings, the database helps those who use it to obtain references pertaining to EA. As an additional research tool and for a nominal fee, CANE has published detailed annotated bibliographies of EA articles and research studies. CANE's goal is to include current web links to these publications, reports, and online training materials; however, some references, such as books, manuals, or videos, must be obtained directly from the publisher or producer. Whenever possible, contact and pricing information is included within the abstracts. CANE has prepared a number of bibliographies, replete with a citation, abstract, and web link. It also includes a summary of recent work from a variety of disciplines relevant to professional practice in the field.

National Center on Elder Abuse. The NCEA was established in 1988 as a national EA resource center under the aegis of the OAA (passed in 1965) and granted a permanent home at AoA/ACL in the 1992 amendments made to Title II of the OAA (NCEA, 2016). The purpose of the NCEA is to provide relevant information, materials, and support, which enhance state and local prevention and intervention efforts concerning EA. The NCEA disseminates news and resources; collaborates on research; provides consultation, education, training, and information about promising practices and interventions; answers inquiries and requests for information; operates a listserv forum; and advises on program and policy development. As another function, the NCEA facilitates the exchange of strategies for discovering and prosecuting fraud and scams targeted at older adults. Since its inception, the NCEA has operated by drawing upon a multidisciplinary consortium of partners. Over the years, the partners have sought to address provisions in the OAA through various initiatives aiding the country in better addressing EA. As it has matured, the NCEA has emerged as a critical resource for diverse professionals and academics, as well as national, state, and local aging networks; APS; law enforcement; healthcare professionals; domestic violence networks; and others (Administration for Community Living, 2016).

In 2011, the University of California, Irvine's (UCI)'s Center of Excellence on Elder Abuse and Neglect received an award to serve as NCEA's Information Clearinghouse (Administration for Community Living, 2016). The Clearinghouse is a national information compilation that supports federal, state, and local efforts for prevention, identification, and intervention in situations of EA. In addition, the Clearinghouse offers information and technical support, translates research, and disseminates best practices for state, local, and tribal practitioners. As of this writing, the NCEA and the NCEA Information Clearinghouse is housed at the Keck School of Medicine of the University of Southern California (USC Center on Elder Mistreatment, 2016).

Over time, the scope of NCEA's activities has expanded to include a focus on specific segments of the older adult population. For example, in 2011 first-time funding specifically dedicated to EA prevention in Indian country was awarded to the University of North Dakota (UND). This effort created the NCEA National Indigenous Elder Justice Initiative (NCEA NIEJI). Its efforts to help tribes address EA, neglect, and exploitation include establishing a resource center; identifying and making available existing relevant literature, resources, and tribal codes; and developing and disseminating culturally appropriate and responsive resources for use by tribes, care providers, law enforcement, and other stakeholders.

National Long-Term Care Ombudsman Program. Another program under the umbrella of ACL/AoA is the Long-Term Care Ombudsmen, who are advocates on the local level and work for quality care and treatment for residents of nursing homes, board and care homes, assisted living facilities, and similar adult care facilities (Administration for Community Living, 2016). In particular, Long-Term Care Ombudsmen work to resolve problems of individual residents and to bring about changes at the local, state, and national levels that will improve residents' care and quality of life. The program began in 1972 as a demonstration program that eventually expanded to all states, the District of Columbia, Puerto Rico, and Guam as authorized by the OAA. Each state has an Office of the State Long-Term Care Ombudsman, which is headed by a full-time state ombudsman who directs the work of thousands of local ombudsman staff and volunteers. The statewide programs are federally funded under Titles III and VII of the OAA as well as other federal, state, and local sources. ACL also funds the National Long-Term Care Ombudsman Resource Center, which provides training and technical assistance to state and local ombudsmen; it is operated by the National Consumers' Voice for Quality Long-Term Care (or Consumer Voice) in conjunction with the National Association of States Agencies on Aging United for Aging and Disabilities (NASUAD).

National Adult Maltreatment Reporting System (NAMRS). The NAMRS project was funded in September 2013 by ACL at $1.2 million, received from the FY 2013 Prevention and Public Health Fund (PPHF). It was initiated by ACL and the Department of Health and Human Services' Office of the Assistant Secretary for Planning and Evaluation (ASPE) in light of the continuing need to gather and compile consistent national data on adult mistreatment (Administration for Community Living, 2016). The goal

RESEARCH BOX

Anthony et al. (2009) discuss the challenges for research and practice in elder mistreatment by pointing out that research studies often fail to include all major types of EA in their investigation, focusing on only one type of abuse, such as neglect or physical abuse, or examining only a few selected types. The authors contend that assessment of elder mistreatment is hindered by a myriad of factors, including inconsistent definitions, divergent and untested theories of causation, and limited research attention to the problem. In addition to these difficulties, professionals encounter complex situations requiring considerable clinical assessment skills and decision-making capacity. The authors believe that the prevalence, incidence, and causes of the various types of elder mistreatment are almost impossible to determine accurately with today's tools. When they use only a list of the major types of EA, APS workers and researchers encounter difficulties in their efforts to identify instances of mistreatment. APS workers, as well as mandated reporters such as healthcare providers and social workers, need an assessment tool that can reliably and accurately assess elder mistreatment.

Anthony et al. introduce six screening instruments that meet their criteria to assess current abuse or risk for future abuse and that have utility in service provision and prevention efforts. The assessment instruments are designed to assess safety; access; cognitive status; emotional status; health and functional status; social and financial resources; and the frequency, severity. and intent of the abuse. On the basis of a structured review of screening and assessment instruments, the article explains the psychometric properties of these instruments and their relevance to APS. Existing screening and assessment instruments tend to focus on indicators of physical abuse and exploitation that are readily observable. Some are not useful if their administration is too lengthy, so brevity accompanied with reliability is critical. Probing for subtle signs of potential neglect or abuse is challenging. Although more prevalent, cases of neglect are exceptionally difficult to assess. Implications of the findings for future research, practice, and policy are also discussed in this article, along with recommendations to promote multidisciplinary approaches to policy and practice.

of the pilot initiative was to design a national system for reporting data on adult abuse using information from state APS agency information systems that, although not capturing all forms of abuse, contain information to help advance public awareness of and broader action to prevent and stop EA. The design of the NAMRS system was informed by input from state agencies, as well as other stakeholders in the field of adult abuse, including the CDC and the DOJ's Bureau of Justice Statistics. NAMRS includes data not only on the abuse of older adults, but also on adults with disabilities.

Centers for Disease Control and Prevention

The operational unit authorized to carry out work to address EA at the CDC is the Division of Violence Prevention (DVP) within the National Center for Injury Prevention and Control (NCIPC) (CDC, 2016). DVP is specifically tasked with the following: (1) providing leadership in developing and executing a national program for the prevention and control of nonoccupational violence-related injuries and death, which addresses EA as one of several forms of interpersonal violence (e.g., youth violence, IPV, sexual violence, suicide, and child abuse and neglect); (2) developing and disseminating policies, recommendations, and guidelines on the prevention of violence such as EA and its consequences; and (3) proposing goals and objectives for national violence prevention and control programs, monitoring progress toward these goals and objectives, and recommending and developing guidelines for priority prevention and control activities (NCIPC Function Statement, available at www.cdc.gov/maso/pdf/NCIPCfs.pdf).

Beyond these initial charges, DVP (1) facilitates strategic planning activities similar to those described earlier by other federal, state, and local agencies, academic institutions, and private and other public organizations; (2) plans, directs, conducts, and supports research focused on the causes of violence such as EA and the development and evaluation of strategies to prevent and control violence-related injuries and deaths; and (3) plans, establishes, and evaluates surveillance systems to monitor national trends in morbidity, mortality, disabilities, and costs of violence-related injuries and deaths, and facilitates the development of surveillance systems by state and local agencies. DVP's efforts to address EA have included work to understand how laws, statutes, and regulations influence efforts to detect and address EA locally in states. The earliest work supported by this division, for example, provided funds to scholars at the University of Iowa who illustrated how variations in definitional content in state legislation translated into differences in what was thought of and responded to as EA (Daly & Jogerst, 2003; Jogerst et al., 2003). These definitional differences also made it challenging to compare or combine estimates of abuse prevalence across states and other jurisdictions because it was verified that different states were not measuring the same behaviors and experiences.

Beyond such policy-focused work, DVP has advanced efforts to address EA using the unique skills, capacities, and capabilities of the public health sector.

One effort intended to create a strong strategic basis for public health that informed work in this area has involved the use of expert panels. These panels make good use of the insights, experiences, and unique perspectives of diverse groups of knowledgeable persons who are intimately acquainted with the challenges and opportunities characterizing work to address EA. The first of such panels (Ingram, 2003) created the agenda for CDC's investments for strengthening efforts to prevent elder mistreatment via the application of the public health approach to violence prevention first used successfully to reduce youth violence, suicide, and IPV (Dahlberg & Mercy, 2009). This agenda concentrated CDC's efforts into the four defining activities of the public health approach: (a) continuously collecting epidemiologic data to help accurately define and monitor trends in the incidence and prevalence of EA; (b) systematically identifying factors, dynamics, and processes that increase and decrease risk of perpetration (i.e., risk and protective factors, influences, and processes); (c) rigorously evaluating practices, programs, policies, and strategies to stop or prevent elder mistreatment by changing its risk and protective factors; and (d) precisely, optimally implementing and spreading effective or promising strategies for its prevention (CDC, 2016).

A second expert panel produced uniform definitions and recommended core data elements for collecting data on EA using a public health surveillance framework. The goal of this effort was to begin eliminating critical conceptual, methodological, and operational barriers. Such barriers prevent the use of different data sources on experiences of EA and hinder achievement of impacts on a population level. This includes being able to reach a space where data on EA can be compiled and analyzed in ways that finally and convincingly answer questions about the true magnitude, scope, and severity of EA as a public health threat.

Definitions and data elements were released by CDC in 2016 after years of work to adequately synthesize insights from the various sectors who care for and about older adults who may experience mistreatment (Hall, Karch, & Crosby, 2016). The release of the uniform definitions and recommended core data elements could be followed by the release of supplementary data elements for use in collecting data on elder abuse within a public health surveillance framework. The supplementary data elements may provide expanded opportunities for use of data from different sectors in ways that enhance understanding of patterns of abuse (Hall, Karch, & Crosby, 2016). This, in turn, could increase knowledge of how prevention strategies should be crafted or altered to stop and prevent elder abuse.

Finally, CDC has supported a limited set of projects focused on achieving methodological improvements in either the collection or use of data on EA. Two of these projects are as follows:

Fatal Elder Maltreatment Surveillance Pilot Project. CDC funded a pilot project linking National Violent Death Reporting System (NVDRS) data with state APS data to capture details of violent death because of EA (Elder Justice Interagency Working Group, 2013, p. 15). It also links "natural" death vital statistics data for the elderly to assist in understanding risk and protective factors for violent death. This project may inform prevention by increasing knowledge about the precursors of violent death and injury as a result of EA.

A Protocol to Inform Development of an Ongoing, Population-Based Survey of Elder Abuse in the United States. To establish and monitor changes and trends in the prevalence and incidence of EA and evaluate the effectiveness of intervention strategies, data must be collected on an ongoing basis. To do this efficiently and effectively, it is crucial that proven EA data collection methods be identified, examined for strengths and weaknesses, and configured to create data collection strategies that can support continuous data collection. As a first step toward this larger goal, CDC supported work to develop a surveillance protocol to inform development of a robust ongoing, population-based survey of EA in the United States. CDC specifically worked with SciMetrika, (www.scimetrika.com), a business that focuses on improving human health, to complete essential foundational tasks to promote survey-based collection of data on EA experiences. The delivered protocol and its supporting products will:

- Assist stakeholders in navigating the survey surveillance implementation process
- Provide comprehensive, evidence-based guidance to inform decision making

- Establish the requirements for carrying out such an endeavor, as well as the factors that may influence successful implementation and sustainability; efforts to finalize the series of products are currently under way

Centers for Medicare and Medicaid Services

The CMS is the agency within the U.S. Department of Health and Human Services charged with the administration of key federal healthcare programs—in particular, Medicare, the federal health insurance program for older adults, and Medicaid, a needs-based, federal/state match program that is a primary payer for nursing home residents requiring such services but who have exhausted their financial resources. As such, CMS has a vested interest in the prevention of abuse, neglect, and exploitation of residents in nursing homes. For example, in the realm of EA prevention, CMS conducts a National Background Check Program that identifies procedures for conducting background checks on all prospective direct-patient-access employees of long-term care facilities and providers (CMS, 2017). Also, CMS has developed programs, including hospice and palliative care, that focus on caregiver and patient support. The CMS website includes free publications and webinars about prevention of EA, such as Program Profiles for EA Prevention, as well as fact sheets that describe CMS programs; present findings on strategies for success, funding, and lessons learned; and describe how each program attends to specific cultural considerations when addressing and preventing EA in tribal communities (CMS, 2016).

Department of Justice

The DOJ represents citizens of the United States in enforcing the law in the public interest and providing protection against criminal activity. The department is made up of 32 offices, boards, divisions, and bureaus with a wide array of functions (DOJ, 2016b). A number of its offices are pertinent to EA. One of these is the research arm of DOJ, the National Institute of Justice (NIJ), situated within the Office of Justice Programs (OJP). NIJ's stated objectives relating to EA are "to identify emerging promising practices and evaluate their effectiveness in improving prevention, detection, and intervention efforts" (NIJ, 2016). For over 10 years, NIJ has solicited rigorous research to investigate and test the effectiveness of EA preventive interventions and has funded over 30 research projects related to the abuse, neglect, and financial exploitation of older adults.

The DOJ also manages and maintains the Elder Justic Initiative (EJI) website, an important resource for victims of EA and financial exploitation and their families, as well as practitioners who serve them, law enforcement agencies and prosecutors, and researchers. The website contains information about how to report EA and financial exploitation in all 50 states and territories; this information can be easily accessed merely by entering a zip code. The website displays three different databases containing sample court pleadings and statutes pertinent for federal, state, and local prosecutors. Also, bibliographic information for thousands of EA and financial exploitation articles and reviews is accessible for persons conducting research. Finally, the website includes resources for practitioners to help prevent EA and assist those who have already been abused, neglected, or exploited (DOJ, 2016a).

NONFEDERAL ENTITIES AND ORGANIZATIONS

Compared with federal organizations, there are a larger number of nonfederal entities and organizations that have sponsored and carried out initiatives, programs, and campaigns to stop and prevent EA. A representative selection of such organizations is described briefly next. The descriptions are intended to provide the reader with an improved awareness of professional and voluntary options for involvement that includes systematic, focused, and well-organized efforts to address EA locally, nationally, and internationally. These organizations are key stakeholders in EA prevention. It is critical that they are engaged as partners with public health to ensure the success of comprehensive, multisectoral efforts to prevent and stop EA.

AARP

AARP, formerly known as the American Association of Retired Persons, is the nation's leading organization for people aged 50 years and older (AARP, 2017). Dr. Ethel Percy Andrus, a retired high school principal, founded AARP in 1958. AARP evolved from the National Retired Teachers Association (NRTA), which Dr. Andrus established in 1947 to promote her philosophy of productive aging and to respond to the need of retired teachers for health insurance. In 1963, Dr. Andrus established an international presence for AARP by founding the Association of Retired Persons International (ARPI), with offices in Lausanne, Switzerland, and Washington,

D.C. Although ARPI disbanded in 1969, AARP has continued to develop networks and form coalitions within the worldwide aging community, promoting the well-being of older persons internationally through advocacy, education, and service. AARP continues to promote independence, dignity, and purpose for older persons; enhance the quality of life for older persons; and encourage older people "to serve, not to be served" (see https://www.aarp .org/about-aarp/company/info-2016/history.html for specifics regarding the history of AARP).

Several of AARP's divisions have services or special programs related to EA. These include the Fraud Fighters Program Kit, Abused Elders or Older Battered Women Report on the AARP Forum, and Survey of Services for Older Battered Women. AARP also assists communities interested in setting up money management and volunteer guardianship programs (see efforts such as those profiled at www.aba.com/Engagement/Pages/AARP.aspx). AARP has been particularly active in launching and supporting educational and awareness efforts to prevent financial exploitation and other forms of EA, and it advocates for elder rights and state-specific needs via a web of AARP state chapters (AARP, 2017). Finally, AARP International has participated in World Elder Abuse Awareness Day (WEAAD), discussed in greater detail later in this chapter.

National Clearinghouse on Abuse in Later Life

The Wisconsin Coalition Against Domestic Violence (see Chapter 6) created the NCALL in 1999 with funding from the DOJ's Office on Violence Against Women (NCALL, 2016). Its mission, to eliminate abuse in later life, is accomplished through advocacy and education. Since 2002, NCALL has provided technical assistance to the DOJ's Office on Violence Against Women for the Enhanced Training and Services to End Abuse in Later Life Program. NCALL is a nationally recognized organization providing leadership on program development, policy, technical assistance, and training that addresses the nexus between domestic violence, sexual assault, and elder abuse, neglect, and exploitation. The organization strives to challenge and change beliefs, policies, practices, and systems that allow abuse to occur and continue. Its focus has helped improve victim safety by increasing the quality and availability of victim services and support. Staff members provide information and resources about programming, outreach, collaboration, and policy development related to abuse in later life and EA. In particular, NCALL staff members provide technical assistance on abuse in later life and respond to questions by phone, email, or in person; they also review materials and participate in state and national advisory committees. Staff and consultants in this organizations train many audiences, including domestic violence and sexual assault programs, aging bureaus, APS, criminal and civil justice system agencies and representatives, healthcare providers, and other legal personnel. NCALL also creates and disseminates a variety of resources and tools on domestic abuse in later life, which are available and searchable on its website (NCALL, 2016).

National Committee for the Prevention of Elder Abuse

The NCPEA is an association of researchers, practitioners, educators, and advocates dedicated to protecting the safety, security, and dignity of America's most vulnerable citizens. Established in 1988, it was founded by Rosalie Wolf to achieve a clearer understanding of abuse and provide direction and leadership to prevent it. For many years, NCPEA was a partner in the NCEA. NCPEA, along with the now defunct MetLife Mature Market Institute, published two highly important and influential documents on elder financial abuse, *Broken Trust* (MetLife Mature Market Institute, National Committee for the Prevention of Elder Abuse, & Center for Gerontology at Virginia Polytechnic institute and State University, 2009) and *The MetLife Study of Elder Financial Abuse: Crimes of Occasion, Desperation, and Predation Against America's Elders* (MetLife Mature Market Institute, National Committee for the Prevention of Elder Abuse, & Center for Gerontology at Virginia Polytechnic Institute and State University, 2011). Currently, NCPEA is engaged in an interdisciplinary national project to explore and address polyvictimization in late life, supported by a grant from the U.S. DOJ, OJP, and Office for Victims of Crime.

International Network for the Prevention of Elder Abuse

With roots in and a continued affiliation with NCPEA, the INPEA was founded in 1997 by EA icon Rosalie S. Wolf (INPEA, 2016). INPEA operates as an independent, nonprofit organization, incorporated under the laws of the Commonwealth of Massachusetts. INPEA functions as a nongovernmental organization (NGO) with special consultative status to the United Nations Economic and Social Council (EcoSoc), UN Department of Economic and Social Affairs (DESA). It is affiliated with the UN Department of Public Information (UN DPI). A member of the Conference of NGOs (Co-NGO), it is composed of regional and national representatives from around the world. INPEA participates in international conferences and research. It is affiliated with numerous organizations, including the African Research Network; Geneva International Network on Ageing; International Association of Gerontology and Geriatrics; Latin America and Caribbean Region IAGG; International NGOs for a Convention on the Human Rights of Older Persons; Institute on Violence, Abuse and Trauma's Annual Conference; National Partnership to End Interpersonal Violence Across the Life Span; and National Initiative on Care of the Elderly (International Network for Prevention of Elder Abuse, 2016).

World Elder Abuse Awareness Day

The World Elder Abuse Awareness Day (WEAAD) is the brainchild of visionary Elizabeth Podnieks of the University of Toronto, and was launched on June 15, 2006, by INPEA and the World Health Organization at the United Nations (INPEA, 2017). The purpose of WEAAD is to provide an opportunity for communities around the world to promote a better understanding of abuse and neglect of older persons by raising awareness of the cultural, social, economic, and demographic processes affecting EA and neglect. In addition, WEAAD supports the United Nations' International Plan of Action, acknowledging the significance of EA as a public health and human rights issue. The annual observance of WEAAD serves as a call to action for individuals, organizations, and communities to raise awareness about EA, neglect, and exploitation (INPEA, 2017).

POLICY BOX

Mixson (2010) examines public policy related to APS in the United States from her perspective of more than 20 years of experience working in a large state APS program and a long-standing involvement in national activities related to EA and adult protection. Mixson writes about her supervisor Paul G. Blanton, a philosopher, social activist, professor, and program specialist in APS, who believed that law should form the skeleton of a program and that program policy written by agency staff should add the flesh that puts the program into effect. Although Blanton acknowledged the ultimate public policy to be law, he held that one written in

(continued)

POLICY BOX (*continued*)

sufficient detail to address the inner operations of a program would be essentially unworkable, because laws, by their nature, and especially in Texas, cannot be amended quickly enough to adjust to and address changes in the "real world," which is the program's frontline environment. Mixson further explains that although basic strategies for addressing the type of abuse can be identified, the personalities, histories, and circumstances of the parties in each protective situation can vary to such a degree that attempting to write policy to fit every circumstance would be futile and counterproductive.

Mixson continues the discussion by emphasizing the importance of building of an infrastructure and the role of ethical practice guidelines, revision, and reporting laws. Questions persist around when, who, and what determines a client's capacity; what constitutes sufficient risk to intervene (whether voluntarily or involuntarily); sharing information at multiple levels (local, state, and interstate); perpetrator registries; the role of APS vis-à-vis guardianship; appropriate supervisor-to-worker ratios; accountability and program evaluation; death reviews; and community involvement, which Mixson regards as the most crucial.

National Adult Protective Services Association

NAPSA is a national nonprofit organization that boasts members in all 50 states. Formed in 1989, NAPSA provides a forum for APS by sharing information, solving problems, and improving the quality of services for victims of elder and vulnerable adult abuse. Its mission is to strengthen the capacity of APS at national, state, and local levels; to effectively and efficiently recognize, report, and respond to the needs of elders and adults with disabilities who are the victims of abuse, neglect, or exploitation; and to prevent such abuse whenever possible (NAPSA, 2017). Currently, NAPSA is engaged in the following activities:

- Operates as the National APS Resource Center to provide APS systems, agencies, and professionals with current and relevant information and support to enhance the quality, consistency, and effectiveness of APS programs across the country

- Partners with diverse organizations to provide a cohesive network of research, practice, and policy to meet the diverse needs of the ever-changing population of vulnerable adults

- Conducts national research on topics such as APS training activities, services to self-neglecting adults, and national APS data collection, as well as partnering with academic researchers on elder and vulnerable adult abuse studies

- Hosts the premier annual national conference on EA as well as a national summit on financial exploitation that features nationally reputable professionals who share their expertise on cutting-edge issues applicable to APS practice and other disciplines

- Works to increase national awareness of elder and vulnerable adult abuse through education, advocacy, and congressional testimony (NAPSA, 2017)

American Bar Association Commission on Law and Aging

Since its inception, the ABA Commission on Law and Aging has been actively engaged in examining a wide range of legal issues affecting older persons (ABA Commission on Law and Aging, 2016). Its mission—to strengthen and secure the legal rights, dignity, autonomy, quality of life, and quality of care of elders—is implemented through research, policy development, technical assistance, advocacy, education, and training. The commission consists of a rotating 15-member interdisciplinary body of national experts in aging and law, including lawyers, judges, health and social services professionals, academics, and advocates. The work of the commission has resulted in policy and practice research and development, coordination and collaboration, education for professional and public audiences, and technical assistance. Over the years, the commission has conducted a number of influential projects and developed publications related to EA and elder rights, including but not limited to those with the following titles: *Capacity Assessment, Dispute Resolution and Mediation, Emeritus Pro Bono, Equal Access to Justice, Ethics and Counseling Older Clients, Guardianship Law and Practice, Healthcare Decision Making, International Rights of Older Persons, Long-Term Care Services and Supports, Medicare,* and *Voting and Cognitive Impairments* (ABA Commission on Law and Aging, 2016).

Safe Havens

Safe Havens is an interfaith organization that promotes hope and justice for victims of domestic violence and EA. Its founder, Anne Marie Hunter, recognized that victims' faith contributed to why they chose to remain in abusive relationships. In 1991, she founded Safe Havens to strengthen the ability of diverse faith communities to respond to victims of domestic violence in Greater Boston (Safe Havens, 2016). Presently, Safe Havens has a national presence and a three-pronged mission to promote safety through faith and entailing awareness (i.e., improving an understanding of the importance and implications of EA to impact attitudes and behavior), advocacy (i.e., uniting people to create a base of public support for social and legislative solutions), and action (i.e., mobilizing forces to prevent elder abuse, neglect, and exploitation).

In addition to Safe Havens, certain religious denominations have addressed EA. For example, the Methodist Church (2000; reaffirmed, 2016) adopted a resolution encouraging church members to take an active stand against the problem. In 2012, the Episcopal Church of the United States passed a resolution at its General Convention addressing EA and includes on its website a Lenten Series of Meditations on the issue (Older Adult Ministries of the Episcopal Church, 2016).

ACADEMIC CENTERS

Academic centers have helped promote and build momentum for efforts to systematically address EA. A number of such centers have not only promoted academic examination and study of EA, but also cultivated advancements in practice and service provision with tangible implications for prevention. Each of the centers highlighted next has contributed to the aforementioned areas in distinctive, notable ways. Moreover, these centers illustrate the use of core public health principles including collaborative, comprehensive coordination of activities by meaningfully involving those who may impact or be impacted by efforts to address the complex, multifaceted population-level problem of EA.

Center for Excellence on Elder Abuse and Neglect

Housed at USC (earlier at UCI) the mission of the Center of Excellence on Elder Abuse and Neglect (CEEN) is to eradicate abuse of older adults. Established by a grant from the Archstone Foundation, CEEN strives to promote aging with dignity and eliminate aging with fear (CEEN, 2016). At the local level, CEEN provides medical, forensic, and victim services to abused and neglected elders living in community or long-term care settings, and thus is a "living laboratory" of innovative approaches. Statewide and nationally, the center serves as a source of technical assistance, multidisciplinary training, useful research, and relevant policy, and, as of 2014, is the administrative home for the NCEA (CEEN, 2016).

Activities of CEEN include/have included the following:

- *Providing direct services*, which include medical assessments, forensic evaluations, and interdisciplinary case planning in partnership with Orange County Adult Protective Services. CEEN is the home of the world's first Elder Abuse Forensic Center, which brings together physicians, psychologists, law enforcement, social workers, and others to handle complex cases of EA and to help keep older adults safe.

- *Giving technical assistance*, including resources related to EA and neglect to assist professionals and the public at large.

- *Conducting research* through the efforts of faculty and partners. CEEN provides a bridge between direct service providers and academics. Research has been funded through the National Institute on Aging, National Institute on Justice, and the California Department of Health and Human Services.

- *Conducting education* through the EA Training Institute, which provides training on issues regarding EA. Multidisciplinary experts conduct discipline-specific training seminars for law enforcement, legal, medical, and social service professionals (CEEN, 2016).

Texas Elder Abuse and Mistreatment Institute

The first collaboration of its kind in the country, the Texas Elder Abuse and Mistreatment Institute (TEAM), was established by Dr. Carmel Dyer, professor and director of the Division of Geriatric and Palliative Medicine and director of University of Texas (UT) Health's Consortium on Aging. Dr. Dyer founded TEAM and led the institute for its first 17 years. She was succeeded by Co-director Jason Burnett, PhD, assistant professor of medicine in the Division of Geriatric and Palliative Medicine.

James Booker, Director of Texas Region VI APS, is also a Co-director of TEAM. TEAM comprises a multidisciplinary group of clinicians, researchers, businesses, social services agencies, APS staff, attorneys, and community groups. Its purpose is to educate healthcare professionals, community services workers, and the public; conduct research; review cases of elder deaths and financial exploitation; and provide clinical care and social and behavioral interventions to abused and neglected elders. Replicated across the United States, the TEAM Institute has received more than $5 million in grants and research funding and has published more than 70 papers, 50 abstracts, four book chapters, and one book (Texas Department of Family and Protective Services, 2016; UTHealth, 2016).

New York City Elder Abuse Center

In 2009, the New York–Presbyterian Hospital/Weill Cornell Medical Center created the New York City Elder Abuse Center (NYCEAC) to improve intervention and treatment for EA cases in the New York City area. The recipient of two grants totaling $375,250 (Weill Cornell Medical College, 2009), NYCEAC is the first center in the New York area to focus on coordinating EA cases.

Mark Lachs, MD, MPH, Co-chief of the Division of Geriatrics and Gerontology, director of the Center for Aging Research and Clinical Care at New York-Presbyterian Hospital/Weill Cornell Medical Center, and Irene F. and I. Roy Psaty Distinguished Professor of Clinical Medicine at Weill Cornell Medical College, is the executive director of the NYCEAC. The center uses a case consultation approach, hosting regular meetings with clinicians, city agencies, and outreach organizations to determine the best approach for each case. NYCEAC began coordinating cases in Brooklyn and then expanded, serving as a training ground and central resource for technical assistance, innovative best practices, multidisciplinary training, research, and policy development in New York City and other parts of the state. Key partners include APS, Jewish Association for Services for the Aged, Geriatric Mental Health Alliance of New York, Kings County's District Attorney's Office, New York City Department for the Aging, New York Legal Assistance Group, Vera Institute of Justice, and the Harry & Jeanette Weinberg Center for Elder Abuse Prevention at the Hebrew Home in Riverdale (Weill Cornell Medical College, 2009).

DISCUSSION BOX

The predominant (and growing) means of keeping the EA issue in the public and private eye is social media, which allows the federal and nonfederal agencies and entities mentioned in this chapter to publicize and raise awareness about this issue with high frequency and at a low cost. First, however, there is a need to introduce EA as a major public health issue in the social media realm and to develop and discuss different ways that social media could be used in raising awareness as well as serving as an effective communication channel in collaborations between federal agencies, nonfederal organizations, and initiatives. Social media have the potential to act as a collaborative investment to nationalize and gradually globalize the fact that EA is a public health problem. Effective collaboration among different sectors is the key to prevent and address this problem.

CASES AND EFFORTS BY INDIVIDUALS

Population-level information is the aggregation of individual experiences. Although the focus of public health is on a population-level characterization of EA impacts, it is critical to understand the plight and circumstances of those personally affected. It is specifically important to understand the scope of the effects of EA and to get a sense of what can be done to ensure that perpetration of EA does not occur or is stopped as early as possible. It is also important to encourage action to prevent and stop the problem. In this section, we highlight notable cases of EA to ground the reader's consideration of EA in the human conditions that influence the implementation of prevention work and then present efforts initiated by individuals as a way of emphasizing that we all can help stop EA by contributing in ways that we are most able.

Mickey Rooney

Long-lived career actor Mickey Rooney was an alleged victim of EA by his own stepchildren, Chris and Christina Abner. Apparently, the alleged wrongdoing continued until he died in April 2014, at which point he was left with only $18,000 to his name (ABC News, 2011). In 2011, and only weeks after his stepson was served with a restraining order accusing him of financial exploitation, Rooney flew to Washington, D.C. Herb Kohl, chairman of the Senate Special Aging Committee, had read press reports concerning a conservator for Rooney who was pursuing EA charges and invited Rooney to testify about his experiences. At the testimony, Rooney explained that he was a victim of EA, a crime that stripped him "of the ability to make even the most basic decisions about my life," and leading to an "unbearable" and "helpless" daily existence (ABC News, 2011). Only when Rooney confided about the abuse to a Disney executive during the filming of *The Muppets* (2011) was anything done about the situation. Rooney's attorneys petitioned the court for a conservator to protect him from further abuse and help recover his assets. The petition stated that the stepchildren forbade the actor's purchasing food or carrying identification. Particularly telling was an account by Hector Garcia, who was brought in by the appointed conservator and who discovered Rooney lying on the ground. Garcia found Rooney's wife, Jan, standing over Rooney and striking him. Garcia, inquiring why she was doing so, Jan replied, "Get used to it. I hit him because that's the only way he learns—by hitting him like a kid." Jan, who now lives with her son, Chris, maintains that she and her son were falsely accused and that "Mickey was a 90-year-old man who was in and out of it mentally and was easily influenced by other people." Rooney's estate provides his wife $100,000 a year from his Screen Actor's Guild pension and Social Security benefits (Baum & Feinberg, 2015).

Brooke Astor/Phillip Marshall

Highly visible philanthropist Brooke Astor was the chairwoman of the Vincent Astor Foundation, established by her third husband, Vincent Astor, son of John Jacob Astor IV and great-great grandson of America's first multimillionaire, John Jacob Astor. Mrs. Astor was the victim of abuse at the hands of her son, Anthony Marshall. Her grandson, Dr. Phillip Marshall, a historic preservationist and associate professor at Roger Williams University, filed a lawsuit removing his father as her guardian and appointing Annette de la Renta (wife of Oscar de la Renta) as the new guardian. *The New York Times* accounts reported that Brooke Astor suffered from a variety of health problems, including Alzheimer's disease and anemia. Dr. Marshall's lawsuit alleged that his father failed to provide for Mrs. Astor by allowing her to live in squalor, reducing the number of physician visits and medications that she needed, and paying himself with income from her estate. Following the change in guardian, Mrs. Astor was moved to Holly Hill, her 75-acre estate, where she died in 2007. Also in 2007, the New York District Attorney announced indictments on criminal charges against Anthony Marshall and attorney Francis X. Morrissey, Jr., related to mishandling Astor's money and a questionable signature on a third amendment to her 2002 will. Anthony Marshall was eventually charged with grand larceny, criminal possession of stolen property, forgery, scheming to defraud, falsifying business records, offering a false instrument for filing, and conspiracy in plundering Astor's $198 million estate. Marshall and Morrissey were both sentenced to 1 to 3 years in prison. Anthony Marshall died at the age or 90 years (*New York Daily News*, 2014).

Dr. Phillip Marshall has continued the fight against EA by launching the public Facebook page *Beyond Brooke*, on which he posts the most up-to-date information possible about activities and initiatives to address EA (Facebook, 2016). In addition, Dr. Marshall travels around the country to help raise the visibility of the issue.

William Mapother

In 2007, Louisville, Kentucky, native William Mapother, who starred in the television series *Lost* and movies such as *World Trade Center, Magnolia*, and *In the Bedroom*, recorded a series of public service announcements for the Kentucky Cabinet for Families and Children that were initially Kentucky-specific but were later made suitable for national television and radio public service announcements (Kentucky Cabinet for Health and Family Services, 2009). In 2009, his recordings became a movie trailer for Elder Abuse Awareness Month, the result of a contract between the NCEA and the Screen Actors Guild. The NCEA also posted the series on its website and television stations across the country have aired them. Mapother continues to keep the issue of EA visible by posting information in a blog and on YouTube (YouTube, 2012).

SUMMARY

In view of the information presented in this chapter, it is clear that, with the assistance of federal and nonfederal agencies and entities, the problem of EA is capturing more and more public attention. However, along with this greater attention is the concomitant need to more effectively communicate that the problem can be successfully prevented. The fact that more people are aware of the problem is a strong testament to the tireless work of advocates, researchers, theorists, practitioners, and elders themselves. The predominant (and growing) means of keeping the issue in the public and private eye is social media, which allows the initiatives, organizations, and efforts mentioned in this chapter to publicize and raise awareness about the issue with high frequency and at low cost. Notable among the newest initiatives are efforts by the investment industry concerning elder financial exploitation (e.g., Wells Fargo), the growing presence of literature and film to depict the problem (e.g., PSAs involving persons such as William Mapother from *Lost*), the explosive growth of WEAAD, and vigilant efforts by the NCEA and tenets of the Elder Justice Act to encourage interagency collaboration at the federal level. Recent and effective venues include websites and webinars that allow groups to coalesce around prevention efforts to raise attention to the fact that EA is a public health issue and needs interdisciplinary approaches to address the problem.

Despite the efforts delineated in this chapter, the field is impacted by a lack of funding to address EA efforts. Funding needs delay sorely needed action to resolve this public health problem. Despite these challenges, the active and robust pockets of effort around the country will likely continue. Moreover, the battle to keep the problem visible will continue to be waged using innovative strategies, tools, and tactics used in initiatives. Collaborative investment in efforts to nationalize and globalize the fact that EA is a public health problem, and to actually act to address it as such, is key to prevention and intervention efforts. Also, educating and training future professionals who work in this area is crucial to this initiative. The areas of education and training are precisely where public health has considerable skill, knowledge, and expertise.

Thought-Provoking Questions

Although there has been increasing attention placed on understanding the dynamics of EA, advancement of public policy and scholarly work has been hampered because much of this work occurs in disciplinary silos (Blowers et al., 2012). Moreover, educating and training future professionals in this area is crucial to this initiative.

1. How can university scholars from various disciplines partner with social services providers, legal professionals, and healthcare educators in the community to enhance the development of a sustainable comprehensive network addressing the prevention of EA?

2. What is the potential role of social media in facilitating the collaboration between different agencies and programs around EA prevention? What is the role of social media in facilitating partnerships between universities and social services providers, legal professionals, and healthcare educators in the community?

3. What steps can be taken to promote the training of future professionals in the field of EA? What needs to be done to encourage universities and academic centers to establish related programs or provide educational trainings?

4. What steps need to be taken or incentives should be used to encourage college students to pursue education that takes into account EA education? If you consider exposing high school students to this problem, what are effective ways to shape their interest to seek further education in this field? Provide example of ways to expose them to the topic.

5. What is the most appropriate role of universities in raising awareness about EA? What about the important role of health educators in each community?

6. What is the role of stakeholders working with the elderly population in the community in identifying and addressing EA? What is the level of engagement related to EA for different stakeholders? How can different stakeholders be engaged to prevent and address EA?

7. How could interventions implemented through service programs and agencies be designed in a way to address EA as a national as well as an international public health problem?

REFERENCES

AARP. (2017). AARP real possibilities. Retrieved from http://www.aarp.org
ABC News. (2011). Mickey Rooney takes stand against elder abuse. Retrieved from http://abcnews.go.com/Health/Wellness/mickey-rooney-speaks-senate-committee-elder-abuse/story?id=13037126
Administration for Community Living. (2016). Elder abuse. Retrieved from http://www.aoa.gov
American Bar Association, Commission on Law and Aging. (2016). What we do. Retrieved from http://www.americanbar.org/groups/law_aging.html

178 ELDER ABUSE AND THE PUBLIC'S HEALTH

Anetzberger, G. (2012). An update on the nature and scope of elder abuse. *Generations, 36*(3), 12–20.

Anthony, E. K., Lehning, A. J., Austin, M. J., & Peck, M. D. (2009). Assessing elder mistreatment: Instrument development and implications for Adult Protective Services. *Journal of Gerontological Social Work, 52,* 815–836. doi:10.1080/01634370902918597

Baum, G., & Feinberg, S. (2015). Tears and terror: The disturbing final years of Mickey Rooney. *Hollywood Reporter.* Retrieved from http://www.hollywoodreporter. com/features/mickey-rooneys-final-years-833325?curator=MediaREDEF

Berger, R., & Piliavin, I. (1976). The effect of casework: A research note. *Social Work, 21*(3), 205–208. doi:10.1093/sw/21.3.205

Blenkner, M., Bloom, M., & Nielses, M. (1972). A research and demonstration project of protective services: 289. *Nursing Research, 21*(3), 280.

Blowers, A. N., Davis, B. H., Shenk, D., Kalaw, K. J., Smith, M., & Jackson, K. (2012). A multidisciplinary approach to detecting and responding to elder mistreatment: Creating a university–community partnership. *American Journal of Criminal Justice, 37,* 276–290. doi:10.1007/s12103-012-9156-4

Center of Excellence on Elder Abuse and Neglect. (2016). About us. Retrieved from http://www.centeronelderabuse.org

Centers for Disease Control and Prevention. (2016). Injury prevention and control: Division of Violence Prevention. Retrieved from http://www.cdc.gov/ violenceprevention/elderabuse/index.html

Centers for Medicare and Medicaid Services. (2016). About CMS. Retrieved from https://www.cms.gov/About-CMS/About-CMS.html

Centers for Medicare and Medicaid Services. (2017). National background check program. Retrieved from https://www.cms.gov/Medicare/Provider-Enrollment -and-Certification/SurveyCertificationGenInfo/BackgroundCheck.html

Dahlberg, L. L., & Mercy, J. A. (2009). History of violence as a public health problem. *Virtual Mentor, 11*(2), 167. Retrieved from: http://virtualmentor.ama -assn.org/2009/02/mhst1-0902.html

Daly, J. M., & Jogerst, G. (2003). Statute definitions of elder abuse. *Journal of Elder Abuse & Neglect, 13*(4), 39–57. doi.org/10.1300/J084v13n04_03

Department of Justice. (2016a). Elder Justice Initiative: Prosecutor resources. Retrieved from https://www.justice.gov/elderjustice/prosecutors

Department of Justice. (2016b). Mission statement. Retrieved from http://govinfo .library.unt.edu/npr/library/status/mission/mdoj.htm

Elder Justice Interagency Working Group. (2013). Participating federal departments and agencies mission statements and agency activities relevant to elder justice. Retrieved from https://www.acl.gov/sites/default/files/programs/2016-09/Agency Descriptions.pdf

Facebook. (2016). Beyond Brooke. Retrieved from https://www.facebook.com/ groups/beyondbrooke/members

Hall, J. E., Karch, D. L., & Crosby, A. (2016). Elder abuse surveillance: Uniform definitions and recommended core data elements. Retrieved from http://www.cdc .gov/violenceprevention/pdf/ea_book_revised_2016.pdf

Ingram, E. M. (2003). Expert panel recommendations on elder mistreatment using a public health framework. *Journal of Elder Abuse & Neglect*, *15*(2), 45–65. doi.org/10.1300/J084v15n02_03

International Network for the Prevention of Elder Abuse. (2016). Welcome to the International Network for the Prevention of Elder Abuse. Retrieved from http://www.inpea.net

International Network for the Prevention of Elder Abuse. (2017). World Elder Abuse Awareness Day. Retrieved from http://www.inpea.net/weaad

Jogerst, G. J., Daly, J. M., Brinig, M. F., Dawson, J. D., Schmuch, G. A., & Ingram, J. G. (2003). Domestic elder abuse and the law. *American Journal of Public Health*, *93*(12), 2131–2136. Retrieved from http://ajph.aphapublications.org/ doi/full/10.2105/AJPH.93.12.2131

Kentucky Cabinet for Health and Family Services. (2009). Kentucky-produced ad on elder abuse prevention to be national movie trailer. Retrieved from http://chfs .ky.gov/news/Kentucky-Produced+Ad+on+Elder+Abuse+Prevention+to+be +National+Movie+Trailer.htm

MetLife Mature Market Institute, National Committee for the Prevention of Elder Abuse, & Center for Gerontology at Virginia Polytechnic Institute and State University. (2009). *Broken trust: Elders, family, and finances*. New York, NY: MetLife Mature Market Institute.

MetLife Mature Market Institute, National Committee for the Prevention of Elder Abuse, & Center for Gerontology at Virginia Polytechnic Institute and State University. (2011). *The MetLife study of elder financial abuse: Crimes of occasion, desperation, and predation against America's elders*. New York, NY: MetLife Mature Market Institute.

Mixson, P. M. (2010). Public policy, elder abuse, and Adult Protective Services: The struggle for coherence. *Journal of Elder Abuse & Neglect*, *22*(1–2), 16–36. doi:10.1080/08946560903436148

National Adult Protective Services Association. (2017). About NAPSA. Retrieved from http://www.napsa-now.org/about-napsa

National Center on Elder Abuse. (2016). About NCEA: Mission statement. Retrieved from http://eldermistreatment.usc.edu/national-center-on-elder-abuse-ncea-usc/ about-ncea

National Clearinghouse on Abuse in Later Life. (2016). About NCALL. Retrieved from http://www.ncall.us/about-ncall

National Institute of Justice. (2016). Office of Justice programs, elder abuse. Retrieved from http://www.nij.gov/topics/crime/elder-abuse/pages/welcome.aspx

New York Daily News. (2014). Anthony Marshall, convicted of looting mother Brooke Astor's fortune, dead at 90. Retrieved from http://www.nydailynews.

com/new-york/anthony-marshall-son-brooke-astor-dead-90-article-1
.2029294

Older Adult Ministries of the Episcopal Church, (2016). Elder abuse. Retrieved from http://www.episcopalchurch.org/files/4_elder_abuse.pdf

Safe Havens. (2016). History of Safe Havens: 25 years of making an impact. Retrieved from http://www.interfaithpartners.org/history

Texas Department of Family and Protective Services. (2016). APS and the TEAM Institute. Retrieved from https://www.dfps.state.tx.us/adult_protection/about_adult_protective_services/team.asp

United Methodist Church. (2008). The book of resolutions of the United Methodist Church 2016. Nashville, TN: United Methodist Publishing House. Retrieved from http://www.umc.org/what-we-believe/abuse-of-older-adults

USC Center on Elder Mistreatment. (2016). National Center on Elder Abuse. Retrieved from http://eldermistreatment.usc.edu/national-center-on-elder -abuse-ncea-usc

U.S. Department of Health, Education, and Welfare. (1966). State letter No. 925. Subject: Four model demonstration projects . . . Services to older adults in the Public Welfare Program. Cited in District of Columbia, 1967. In *Protective services for adults: Report on protective services prepared for the D.C. Interdepartmental Committee on Aging*. Washington, DC: Author.

Weill Cornell Medical College. (2009). Weil Cornell newsroom: NYC first elder abuse center. Retrieved from http://news.weill.cornell.edu/news/2009/08/ nycs-first-elder-abuse-center-created-by-newyork-presbyterianweill-cornell -in-collaboration-with-com

Wolf, R. S. (2000). The nature and scope of elder abuse. *Generations, 24*(2), 6–12.

Wolf, R. (2003). *Elder abuse and neglect: History and concepts*. Washington, DC: National Academies Press. Retrieved from https://www.ncbi.nlm.nih.gov/ books/NBK98805

YouTube. (2012). William Mapother elder justice. Retrieved from https://www .youtube.com/watch?v=2vOXtCVfqTA

8

PUBLIC HEALTH, HUMAN RIGHTS, AND GLOBAL PERSPECTIVES ON ELDER ABUSE

Elizabeth Podnieks and Cynthia Thomas

Although the domains of public health and human rights overlap, effective interventions in instances of elder abuse (EA) may be hindered by the lack of an integration of human rights principles in healthcare (Mercy, Butchart, Rosenberg, Dahlberg, & Harvey, 2008). This chapter addresses issues of civil and human rights of all older people, regardless of sexual orientation, ethnicity, or socioeconomic status, toward a future free from EA. The authors argue that elder mistreatment can be addressed more effectively than it is nowadays, and that technology provides tools to enhance both detection and prevention techniques. Grounded in a dynamic public health model of elder mistreatment, research can provide the underpinning for advances in this area. The chapter reviews the history of the recognition of EA as a problem in Canada and the United States, and summarizes the progress to date in dealing with EA in six public health systems around the world. The authors believe that it is possible for people to experience a just society as they grow older—one in which there is recognition of the right to equal opportunity and just treatment in all aspects of life (Perel-Levin, 2008).

Chapter Objectives

By the end of this chapter, readers will be able to

- Understand the connections between public health, human rights, and EA.

- Learn about the progress and limitations in dealing with EA in selected countries.

- Describe potential uses of technology in addressing EA.

- Identify research needs in the field of EA.

Population aging is, first and foremost, a success story for public health policies as well as social and economic development. Population aging is one of humanity's greatest triumphs and also one of its greatest challenges. Although considerable attention is focused on the increased economic and social demands placed on all countries by aging populations, there is little acknowledgment of older people as valuable members of society and persons contributing crucial knowledge, experiences, and expertise to their families and communities. Instead, in many countries around the world, older people and their vital contributions are often overlooked and ignored; too many of them face abuse. The context for this chapter flows from the World Health Organization (WHO) *Report on Violence and Health* (2002) and the WHO 2014 *Global Status Report on Violence Prevention*.

The purpose of this chapter is to engage the reader in exploring and embracing the critical link between EA as an important public health issue and human rights. Seventy years ago, the United Nations (UN) adopted the Universal Declaration of Human Rights (UDHR, 1948) to guarantee all human beings security, dignity, and well-being in every country of the world. Health professionals have a particular stake in the UDHR because human rights and health concerns share the common goals of alleviating suffering and promoting the conditions for health and well-being of all people. There are many connections between health and human rights, across all age cohorts and for older adults in particular. For example, discrimination against older adults, including those who are members of ethnic, religious, and racial minorities, as well as those of a particular gender, sexual orientation, immigration status, or political opinion, compromises or threatens health and well-being, and even the lives of many elderly persons. Discriminatory practices threaten physical and mental health and may deny people actual access to care, therapies, and treatments. Abused elders subjected to discrimination may face an even greater lack of understanding and support for their precarious plight. Respect for human dignity is an essential element of health and well-being of all people—in other words, a human right.

In this chapter, after a discussion of the importance of human rights to public health practices, a schematic public health model is presented and explained, emphasizing the connection between sound public health practices and the promotion of public awareness, detection, and treatment of EA. The discussion then focuses on an overview of the history of the recognition of EA as an important problem first in the United States and then in Europe, followed by an examination of the progress in addressing EA in several international jurisdictions—namely, the Czech Republic, Dominican Republic, Spain, Nepal, Israel, and Quebec, Canada.

Canada's public health programs, which were designed in the 1970s but continue to evolve, are examined as potential templates for other countries. This examination is followed by a description of the current boom in information and communication technologies (ICT), which provide promising opportunities for promoting health as well as for detecting and preventing EA. Communication technologies are becoming powerful tools in the creation, dissemination, and sharing of ideas for building safe, healthy communities worldwide in unprecedented ways (Ranck, 2012). A call for further research and evaluation of the uses of these powerful tools to advance the public health agenda concludes the chapter.

HUMAN RIGHTS AND PUBLIC HEALTH WORKING TOGETHER

Without health, other rights have little meaning.
—World Health Organization

The past decade has led to an increased awareness of the close connection between public health and human rights, and of their complementary roles in violence prevention. This awareness has led to the development of more training programs for health professionals. Schools of medicine, public health, nursing, social work, and gerontology have inaugurated full courses, short courses, conferences, and webinars to promote understanding and knowledge about the relationship between healthcare and human rights. In affirming and supporting human rights, practitioners in all fields of health enhance the ethics of their professions and reinforce their commitments to promoting physical and mental wellness. When human rights are protected, health is improved. If individuals are treated in ways that meet their needs, they are empowered to lead healthier lives and, collectively, the overall level of health of the public is improved (Mann et al., 1994).

> *Respect is better than food or drink.*
> —World Health Organization and International
> Network for the Prevention of Elder Abuse, 2002

The human rights theme is emergent in the EA literature. There is, however, a continuing debate on the need for joining public health and human rights to ensure an equitable society in which older people are valued and cared for in a respectful and dignified manner, despite the declaration by the UN in 1991 that older adults are entitled to the protection of their rights and fundamental freedoms, including full respect for their dignity, beliefs, needs, and privacy. A human rights framework and its attendant freedoms underpin a clear understanding of elder mistreatment across the globe. Attaining one's highest level of physical, social, and mental health, as well as being free from harm, is recognized as a human right.

A central component of human rights is respect for the individual: A respectful approach to elder mistreatment means that older people are recognized and acknowledged for having "a voice" in defining what they perceive as mistreatment and determining how the mistreatment will be addressed. This rights perspective represents a significant paradigm shift away from a "patronizing," "expert" approach—one in which healthcare or other providers presume to know what is best when mistreatment has occurred and the most appropriate interventions are to be chosen. A touchstone of respect is the acknowledgment and celebration of the uniqueness of each person (Perel-Levin, 2008). The healthcare professional's role changes from that of expert to advisor, providing an older person with the best available information and advice at the time to facilitate that person's wishes, and protecting vulnerable

---

DISCUSSION BOX

Older adults' lives can be affected by important ethical issues similar to those faced by adults of all ages. Discuss how service providers may struggle with questions about the following aspects of care:

- The best way to help people in distress

- How to respect personal choices

(continued)

- Is there a limit to the choices older people should be allowed?

- Ethical issues in healthcare treatments

- The scope of ageism

- The importance of cultural values and beliefs held by older adults

- Maintaining the quality of life at the end of life

individuals. This approach creates a culture of inclusion for all, regardless of health status, or economic or social levels.

Within a human rights framework, the responsibilities of leadership, in governments, industries, and other organizations, are defined in terms of how resources can be used to ensure individual safety and well-being, free from paternalism. Questions such as how resources will be dispensed, and to whom, should be scrutinized through a human rights filter so that every person is free from harm and from condescension. A human rights perspective begins at the individual level and expands to communities, society at large, and, ultimately, to nations around the globe (Columbia University Mailman School of Public Health, 2009).

The concept of elder mistreatment in relation to human rights has often been ignored by researchers and policy makers, and indeed by older people themselves. Flynn (2005) suggests that healthcare professionals often have a poor understanding of the relationship between human rights and the guiding principles of nursing care. The challenge is to implement a perspective in which theory and practice merge. Such an approach will demand creative thinking, especially when operationalized with "fringe" or vulnerable populations that are marginalized—immigrants, refugees, people with disabilities, Aboriginal persons, visible minorities, and lesbian, gay, bisexual, transgender, and questioning (LGBTQ) communities.

HUMAN RIGHTS FOR VULNERABLE POPULATIONS

If the goal of public health is "good health for all," then such a goal begs a question: How is a human rights lens best applied to how abuse is prevented, detected, and treated among people who are already stigmatized and who may have internalized societal shame as they age and move into retirement communities, nursing homes, and hospitals? Individuals are at the center of a human rights approach, so they should be encouraged to guide their own lives. How do institutions implement human rights practices and what might those practices look like? These are the questions that drive new thinking in how EA is detected and treated, particularly for diverse populations in a variety of settings. Consider, for example, rules and policies in many institutions regarding meal and bathing times for patients or clients. Policies often are designed for the convenience of staff or in compliance with regulations, with little or no flexibility to accommodate the preferences of the individuals being served.

Such intractable treatment is magnified for marginalized populations. For example, the social exclusion experienced by LGBTQ communities has been described as both emotional abuse and societal abuse (Ploeg, Lohfeld, & Walsh, 2013). Harrowing stories exist about aging LGBTQ persons in both long-term care and home care settings where exclusion, humiliation, and indignity are part of the daily landscape. According to Harrison and Riggs (2006), many older LGBTQ persons live in fear of having their identities revealed and of not being allowed to continue long-term relationships. Any sign of affection between gay or lesbian couples living in long-term facilities can easily cause conflict and may even result in ongoing discrimination and expressions of homophobia, both of which contribute to and exacerbate elder mistreatment, in violation of human rights, and of huge concern for public health (Cook-Daniels, 1997). Consequently, care providers must be on high alert to further understand the needs of this population and adapt interventions accordingly. It is reassuring that the 2015 White House Conference on Aging included major breakthrough recommendations to ensure that LGBTQ voices would be heard. These recommendations are further strengthened by the ongoing movement that aims to foster dialogue and civil engagement around the creation of a new UN Convention on the Rights of Older Persons.

A recent U.S. national study on LGBT health found that 82% of members of the LGBT community experienced victimization (SAGE, 2015). The most common type of victimization was verbal insults (68%), followed by threats of physical violence (43%) and being hassled by police (27%). It is estimated that 1.5% of older Americans identify as LGBT; this number could actually be 3 million and growing. There is no reason to believe that the types of victimization experienced in the United States are any less common in other countries around the world. According to study cited by David Tenenbaum (2012), members of the LGBT community everywhere experience higher rates of victimization, which crime statistics underestimate because people are reluctant to go to the police.

A webinar conducted by NYCEA Elder Justice Dispatch (January, 2014) reported a visionary, important step toward making sure that LGBT older persons in the United States are properly assessed in the Medicaid long-term care system and receive the best patient-centered care possible. State agencies are addressing some of the barriers and health disparities that often face the LGBT population by developing procedures that could potentially improve the coordination of care and service delivery by evaluating individual health status, needs and preferences. Simple changes in the way that providers approach older persons in asking about LGBT identities can result in older adults feeling comfortable enough to discuss discrimination and abuse (Cruz, 2014). On a cautionary note, it is incumbent on healthcare providers—or indeed, any persons in positions of power—to truthfully examine their own feelings and attitudes toward marginalized people: If the compassion is not there, then it is an ethical responsibility to work with other populations or in other settings.

CODIFYING HUMAN RIGHTS FOR OLDER ADULTS

Fredvang and Biggs (2012) discuss the perception of aging as a social problem built on the assumption that older persons are separate from those who are not old—that the aged and the nonaged are two different categories of human beings. Older persons are often seen as nonproductive and thus unable to contribute to society—the perceived "burden" of older persons reinforces their marginality. The impact of advances in health and longevity were not foreseen when the first international human rights instruments were developed. As a result, older people's rights were not explicitly codified. The lack of explicit reference to older people in international law is a glaring omission that advocates are attempting to address now.

Advocates for drafting a new Convention on Human Rights point out that the human rights of older persons are being violated. When older persons suffer specific forms of abuse, such as age discrimination, the right to earn an income, access to justice, or lack of healthcare or housing, they then deserve specific protections similar to those granted to other disadvantaged groups such as people with disabilities. There is little in international rights law that addresses these types of abuse of older people, depriving them of their dignity and causing a protection gap. The adoption of a new Convention would reduce the marginalization of older people, increase their social inclusion, and help eliminate disadvantages specifically associated with later life (Fredvang & Biggs, 2012).

CONCEPTUAL FRAMEWORK FOR ELDER ABUSE AND PUBLIC HEALTH

A dynamic, multidimensional international conceptualization of EA—its causes, manifestations, and consequences—is easily grounded in a public health framework, reinforced by considerations of human rights for all older populations. Under the leadership of the WHO, with six regional offices in Africa, the Americas, Southeast Asia, Europe, the Eastern Mediterranean, and the Western Pacific, and supported by the World Bank and United States Agency for International Development, public health concepts have achieved universal and international recognition, even though they are not always accompanied by a similar dedication to principles of human rights. According to WHO (1998, p. 3), public health is defined as "the art and science of preventing disease, prolonging life, and promoting health through the organized efforts of society."

Although the definition of public health is widely accepted, particular countries focus on different public health issues, according to such factors as their stage in economic development, and poverty levels of the population. Cultural and religious differences, however, make respect for human rights problematic in certain countries, and especially problematic for the rights of women, religious and ethnic minorities, and the elderly.

Developing countries are primarily concerned with infectious diseases, including malaria and tuberculosis, and need to build and improve basic infrastructures such as hospitals, water supply systems, and sanitation (Macfarlane et al., 2000). In Africa, for example, effective prevention efforts are lacking for many diseases, and treatments often cannot keep up with new infections (Cooke, 2009). In Europe and North America, infectious diseases are more often under control, and chronic conditions such as heart disease and cancer are the primary focus of public health efforts. Regardless of the level of poverty or stage in development, nations worldwide recognize EA as a public health problem, whether they are able to cope with it effectively, and regardless of varying culturally determined definitions as to what constitutes abuse.

FRAMEWORKS FOR ELDER ABUSE

As pointed out by the National Council on Ageing and Older People (1998), there are a variety of frameworks for understanding EA. A legal framework has the purpose of identifying appropriate interventions by authoritative sources such as executive and judicial bodies. A case management framework provides a basis for identifying a person's eligibility for services. A framework developed for research purposes can facilitate the study of causal relationships and lead to explanations of behaviors. A public health framework would likely include at least two of these dimensions and should facilitate a better understanding of the dynamics, leading ultimately to prevention.

Generally, explanatory models have been limited to a particular nation or culture. One of the most ambitious, a "schematic outline" presented by Bonnie and Wallace (2003, pp. 62–63), focuses on the sociocultural context of maltreatment, including status inequality, power, and exchange dynamics across regions, states, urban versus rural localities, institutions, and ethnic and racial groups. However, the framework was developed from a Western rather than a cross-cultural perspective. Outcomes specified by the Bonnie and Wallace model emphasize physical and emotional aspects of abuse rather than prevention, the most important emphasis on public health. The schema is intended to provide direction to future researchers more so than to guide any policy development or practices.

Mercy, Rosenberg, Powell, Broome, and Roper (1993) put forward a practical approach to identifying and preventing violence that could include elder abuse, but couched it in the form of a static, rather than a dynamic, model. The model specified three steps leading to the implementation of interventions: defining the problem, identifying causes, and developing and testing interventions. Given that public health issues associated with EA are likely to be constantly evolving with each cohort of elders, with new approaches fostering public awareness, methods of detection enhanced by developments in technology, new treatment strategies, and ultimately new ways to prevent abuse, the model must be dynamic, allowing for feedback and changes over time.

A DYNAMIC PUBLIC HEALTH MODEL OF ELDER ABUSE

A public health model of EA should include elements of promotion of awareness by the general public as well as professionals (including education, training, media campaigns, and use of the Internet), detection (processes by which relevant authorities are informed that an alleged incident of abuse has taken place), and development of laws and regulations that support intervention and treatment strategies. Disease prevention is an important public health objective, and preventing EA (primary prevention) as well as recognizing it (secondary prevention) and "treating" it when it occurs (tertiary prevention) is essential to the well-being of vulnerable older persons.

The specific elements of such a model remain to be "tested" to discover, for example, how well various types of public awareness programs lead to detection and how detecting abuse can be followed up by successful treatments and interventions. It is critical to ascertain which components and types of activities and treatments are most effective in achieving the ultimate goal of preventing the abuse and neglect of elders. To this end, such a public health model must borrow from and incorporate elements from the explanatory factors hypothesized in other models—the risk factors that facilitate abuse, which include characteristics of the older person (e.g., frailty, dementia,) or of the environment (especially, isolation) or the presence of family members with mental illness or substance abuse problems (Lachs, Williams, O'Brien, Hurst, & Horwitz, 1997). Issues associated with EA are most appropriately incorporated in a public health framework; such a conceptualization is an important tool for policy development. To date, no such universal tool has been developed, although numerous researchers and practitioners have attempted to explore and explain various attributes of EA. A schematic form of a dynamic public health model is shown in Figure 8.1, incorporating culture-free elements that can be applied universally.

PERCEPTIONS AND PRACTICES OF ELDER ABUSE: UNITED STATES

EA has not always been perceived as a public health issue or as a violation of human rights. Indeed, the human rights of elders as well as EA itself have long been perceived as secondary in importance to child abuse. In the

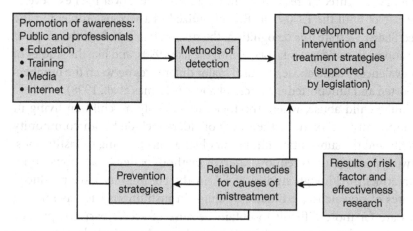

Figure 8.1 Dynamic model of elder abuse prevention

United States, for example, child abuse received national attention as a serious crime as early as the 1930s, when it was recognized under the first Social Security Act (SSA). For the next several decades, however, even though it was considered an important problem, "battered child syndrome," as it was known, was regarded as an infrequent phenomenon and so little was done to address it. As more evidence of its existence came to public attention, legislation supporting the investigation of child abuse was finally passed in the 1950s under amendments to the SSA, and elders were also included in the same legislation although actual programs concerning the investigation of the abuse of children were developed first.

Under the SSA amendments, states were required to fund programs to protect children from abuse and neglect through child protection agencies. Congress also provided funds under the 1950 act to set up protective services units to respond to reports of abuse and neglect of adults and elders, modeling these units after the child protection agencies. Although the legislation covered both child abuse and abuse of adults, children remained the dominant focus of public policies and concerns. U.S. policy makers thought it important to understand the magnitude of the child abuse problem well before paying serious attention to EA. One possible reason for the greater concern for children over older adults is that the experience of childhood is universal, but old age remains a mystery to younger people (Marsh, 2003). Under the Child Abuse Prevention and Treatment Act (CAPTA) of 1974, a National Center on Child Abuse and Neglect was established, and a "full and complete" study of the problem was authorized for the first time. The first national study of the incidence of child abuse was undertaken in 1979, revealing that only a minority of abused and neglected children were reported to official sources (Sedlak, 1991). Three more such studies were conducted over the next several decades. Not until the 1970s was EA recognized as a serious problem in the United States. Despite this recognition, the first national study of the scope of abuse and neglect did not take place until the late 1990s, and like the studies of the prevalence of child abuse, it found major differences between the numbers of reported and unreported instances of abuse (Thomas et al., 1998).

Unlike child abuse, where the focus was mainly on children living in the community, concern for the safety of elders included both community residents and the substantial number of older adults residing in institutions. The two types of settings require different methods of detection, prevention, and treatment. Although studies of EA in the community have produced estimates of prevalence, estimates of abuse in institutions such as nursing homes are far more difficult to obtain because of access barriers, privacy regulations, and the large numbers of adults in residence with dementia and frailty who are less able to provide information about their treatment. Nonetheless, studies have substantiated the fact that abuse is ongoing and remains prevalent, both in community settings and in nursing homes and other group residences, with rates among community-dwelling elders estimated as high as 7.6% to 10.0 % in the United States (Acierno et al., 2010; Cooper, Selwood, & Livingston, 2008; Pillemer & Finkelhor, 1998; Thomas, 2000).

PERCEPTIONS AND PRACTICES OF ELDER ABUSE: EUROPE

Recognition of EA as a societal problem was even slower to take root in Europe than in the United States. Similar to the United States, child abuse was recognized as a problem first, but considerably later than in the United States. In Ireland, for example, the constitution (Article 41, 1937) establishes the family as a "fundamental unit group of society" and superior to "all positive law," implying that attention should be paid to protecting members of families. However, not until 1991 was a Child Care Act passed that required health boards to identify children who were not receiving adequate care in their homes. Two years later, an incest case sparked nationwide concern about child abuse. Similar levels of concern for older adults were minimal until 1998, when a report was published that called attention to the need for legal protections for older adults. The report led to a series of commissions and proposals for legislation on the abuse and neglect of elderly people. Despite increased attention to this issue, as of 2015, no specific legislation on EA had been passed.

Progress in the rest of Europe parallels the Irish experience. However, unlike in many other nations outside Europe, a linkage was made between human rights and EA. Generally, most cases of EA in Europe are treated under human rights or domestic violence legislation, although this legislation does not specifically address older adults (Georgantzi, 2012).

PREVALENCE STUDIES

Policy makers and legislators often want to know that a problem is serious before taking action. Research identifying the scope of the problem of EA was limited until quite recently. Estimates of prevalence vary widely, at least in part because of widely divergent definitions and methodologies of measurement and sampling. An early study in the Netherlands (1998) found a prevalence rate of 5.6% across various forms of EA. Since then, other studies have suggested that the magnitude of the problem is large enough to warrant serious attention by policy makers (Acierno et al., 2010; Comijs, Pot, Smit, Bouter, & Jonker, 1998; Cooper et al., 2008; Thomas, 2000). In 2002, the Madrid International Plan of Action on Ageing (MIPAA) identified EA as a serious concern and received international attention, although the implementation of constructive responses was slow. In 2010, the European Reference Framework Online for the Prevention of Elder Abuse Project (EuROPEAN) included information from 11 countries represented by 77 experts on the awareness of and attention to issues of EA among public health professionals and others in their countries. Despite the promise of the MIPAA in calling attention to the issue, experts noted that specific legislation dealing with EA did not yet exist in any of the 11 nations (Austria, Germany, Greece, Ireland, Italy, Poland, Portugal, Czech Republic, the Netherlands, Slovenia, and Slovakia).

A recent study of the prevalence of five categories of abuse across seven European cities—Stuttgart, Germany; Athens, Greece; Ancona, Italy; Kaunas, Lithuania; Porto, Portugal; Granada, Spain; and Stockholm, Sweden—estimated that rates of psychological abuse, the most common form, ranged as high as 29.7% in Sweden and 10.4% in Italy (Lindert, J., de Luna, Torres-Gonzales, Barros, & Ioannidi-Kopolou, 2013). In contrast, estimates in the United States range from 2% to 10%.

PROGRESS IN ADDRESSING ELDER ABUSE IN SIX COUNTRIES

With the exception of Japan, Asian and African countries also have been slow to develop research, pass legislation, and create programs to prevent and treat EA (Ferreira, 2008). Many developing countries are heavily invested in promoting public awareness through media campaigns and other forms of publicity, but have few laws and regulations governing detection and intervention. Nonetheless, awareness is increasing around the globe, and private organizations and governments have taken steps to address the issues with varying degrees of success. A sampling of progress from selected countries on the basis of recent reports from prominent academics and practitioners is presented in Table 8.1. These countries are located in several different regions of the world—Central America, Europe, Eastern Europe, the Middle East, and Asia; the data also include a country's province in North America. Although not necessarily representative of these regions, they provide a diverse snapshot of ongoing activities and innovations.

Some countries have relatively weak public health programs that are supplemented by the activities of private organizations (e.g., Nepal,

TABLE 8.1 PROGRESS DEALING WITH ELDER ABUSE: PUBLIC HEALTH SYSTEMS IN SIX COUNTRIES

	Core Competencies of Public Health	Barriers and Gaps to Dealing Effectively with Elder Abuse	Promising Practices and Successes
Czech Republic	Regulations and rules for care and treatment of elderly people have been established	Failure to comply with rules due to lack of money Limited staff to carry out policies Low salaries discourage professionals and others from participating Unlicensed facilities provide inadequate care	The media are active in reporting cases of abuse The Government Council for Seniors receives complaints of abuse The Czech ombudsman reports complaints to the police
Dominican Republic	The National Council of Ageing People—not the Ministry of Public Health—is responsible for establishing policies regarding awareness, prevention, and treatment of elder abuse	The National Council has been unable to develop an effective system for reporting, intervention, and treatment Mistreated elders must report abuse to the Department of Interfamilial Violence but often are afraid to do so Even when the National Council brings a perpetrator to justice, there is often no follow-up for the victim	Increasing press coverage of awareness events The public defender has been sensitized to the issues Establishment of a 24-hour hotline

TABLE 8.1 PROGRESS DEALING WITH ELDER ABUSE: PUBLIC HEALTH SYSTEMS IN SIX COUNTRIES (*continued*)			
	Core Competencies of Public Health	Barriers and Gaps to Dealing Effectively with Elder Abuse	Promising Practices and Successes
Spain	The Organization, Autonomy, and Care of Dependent Adults (SAAD) was established after passage of Public Law 39/2006 in January 2007 with the collaboration of public and private agencies State Reference Centers have been established by the Spanish Ministry of Health as a system of services for the autonomy and care of dependent adults Over 10 programs coordinated by private and governmental organizations serve elderly persons who may be the victims of abuse or neglect	Although the crime of habitual family violence was formally established in 1989, there is no specific law regulating elder abuse	Various public awareness programs: • Ponte en su ("Put yourself in their shoes") • World Elder Abuse Awareness Day • Alzheimer's program • Juntos Podemos ("Together we can") • Matradoa personas mayores ("Elder abuse") Training for Professionals under Article 36, Law 39/2006 A royal decree recognizing nonprofessional caregivers An innovative elder security plan focusing on prevention and improved security for older adults (Plan Mayor de Seguridad)

(*continued*)

TABLE 8.1 PROGRESS DEALING WITH ELDER ABUSE: PUBLIC HEALTH SYSTEMS IN SIX COUNTRIES *(continued)*

	Core Competencies of Public Health	Barriers and Gaps to Dealing Effectively with Elder Abuse	Promising Practices and Successes
Nepal	Ageing Nepal was established in 2011 in affiliation with the Social Welfare Council to take proactive measures against abuse and exploitation of elders	There are barriers to receiving old age assistance, including governmental irregularities Elders are abused and killed due to allegations of witchcraft	Awareness is increasing because of reports in the print and electronic media; actions of government, social, and professional organizations; and contributions from the arts Examples include radio and TV talk shows; articles in newspapers, in magazines, and on Internet blogs; dramas, songs, videos, and pamphlets and posters; and participation in World Elder Abuse Awareness Day
Israel	The Law of Protection of the Helpless (1989) provides a basis for countering elder abuse	Need to establish a better division of responsibility between health and welfare systems and the police and legal system	The Ministry of Welfare and its partners began programs for abuse prevention first in selected municipalities and then in every Welfare Municipal Office

TABLE 8.1 PROGRESS DEALING WITH ELDER ABUSE: PUBLIC HEALTH SYSTEMS IN SIX COUNTRIES (*continued*)

	Core Competencies of Public Health	Barriers and Gaps to Dealing Effectively with Elder Abuse	Promising Practices and Successes
	The Ministry of Health (2003) required health facilities to establish committees headed by social workers to receive reports of elder abuse in community clinics, hospitals, and long-term care organizations, and then to inform the Ministry of Health	Increased development and implementation of professional interventions are needed More training is required for police and courts, if their role is to be increased	The project includes collaboration between the Center for the Prevention of Domestic Violence and the Welfare Department for the Elderly; units include a social worker as the coordinator, a paraprofessional, an advising physician, and a legal expert A special model for intervention was developed for rural councils to deal with economic exploitation of parents because of laws allowing only one son to inherit agricultural holdings
Quebec, Canada	Establishment of the Quebec Human Rights Commission in 1976	Changes in priorities under different ministries Difficulties in addressing elder abuse in institutions	Public awareness An annual public awareness campaign; TV campaign won a prize for its impact University chair on abuse of older adults, involved in over 40 research projects in past 5 years

(continued)

TABLE 8.1 PROGRESS DEALING WITH ELDER ABUSE: PUBLIC HEALTH SYSTEMS IN SIX COUNTRIES (*continued*)

	Core Competencies of Public Health	Barriers and Gaps to Dealing Effectively with Elder Abuse	Promising Practices and Successes
	Development of the Quebec Governmental Action Plan, 2010–2015, by 13 ministries: A collaboration among health and social services, status of women, immigration, education, justice, and public safety organizations aimed at improving services		Detection: Hotline staffed by trained professionals Intervention, treatment, and prevention strategies • Action plans developed by 19 regional coordinators • Publication of a reference guide for prevention, detection, intervention and coordination • Teams of crime prevention officers and social or medical practitioners • Tool box under development for prevention and detection

Information in this table is based on the following contributions:

Lorman, J. (2015). *Czech Republic: Zivot 90, elder mistreatment in the Czech Republic.* Unpublished manuscript.

Pereyra, R. (2015). Dominican Republic: Elder mistreatment and the public's health (unpublished communication from the author).

Iborra, I., Garcia, Y., & Grau, E. (2013). Spain: Public health and elder mistreatment in Spain. In A. Phelan (Ed.), *International perspectives in elder abuse* (pp. 168–187). London, UK: Routledge.

Magar, S. T. & Gurung, A. (2015). Year book of senior citizens 2016. Battisputali, Kathmandu, Nepal: Ageing Nepal. Retrieved from http://ageingnepal.org/wp-content/uploads/2016/02/Final-year-book-2016.pdf

Lowenstein, A. (2015). Israel: President, Max Stern Yezreel Valley College (unpublished communication from the author).

Canadian Network for the Prevention of Elder Abuse. (2017). New Quebec government action plan to counter elder mistreatment (2017–2022) – "Québec keeps innovating". Interview with Marie Beaulieu [Transcript]. Retrieved from https://cnpea.ca/en/about-cnpea/blog/745-new-quebec-government-action-plan-to-counter-elder-mistreatment-2017–2022-québec-keeps-innovating

Czech Republic, and Dominican Republic). All face barriers or gaps in their old age programs either with regard to the absence of the availability of basic benefits (Nepal), failure to enforce regulations related to EA (Czech Republic), lack of specific legislation for regulating EA (Spain), or the need for clarifying policies (Israel). All six report promising practices and successes, particularly with regard to increasing awareness through the media, participation in events such as World Elder Abuse Awareness Day (WEAAD), contributions from the arts, and the distribution of pamphlets and posters. Although fostering awareness has been an important component of the activities in all five countries plus one provincial area, significant barriers remain to dealing effectively with EA, and public policies and laws often are limited.

CANADA'S PUBLIC HEALTH SYSTEM

Among developed nations, Canada has been among the most active in addressing EA in a public health framework supported by an attention to human rights. (Note: The World Trade Organization takes the lead in defining "developed" and "developing"—terms that are still in use.) Public Health Agency of Canada is the federal department responsible for helping Canadians maintain and improve their health while respecting individual choices and circumstances. It is guided by provisions of the Canada Health Act of 1984 and provides universal coverage for medically necessary healthcare on the basis of need. The Canadian model of population health is built on a long tradition of national programs in public health, community health, and health promotion. Good health is regarded as a capacity or resource for everyday living, allowing individuals to pursue goals, acquire skills and education, and grow and attain individual aspirations. The Canadian approach to public health recognizes that many interrelated factors and conditions contribute to overall health. These factors are referred to as "the social determinants of health". Canadian contributions to the social determinants of health started in the 1970s and have been so extensive as to make Canada a "health promotion powerhouse" in the eyes of the international health community. The aim of Public Health Agency of Canada is to preserve and improve the health of all Canadians while reducing health disparities among certain population groups such as immigrants, Native peoples, and people with disabilities. By considering the entire range of evidence-based factors, conditions, and interactions that influence health, improvements in health can be achieved. The Canadian population-based public health approach contributes to overall societal development and ultimately requires less healthcare than a reactive model of public health, while being sustaining and self-supporting over the long term. A population health approach in Canada includes a focus on the interrelated conditions and factors that influence the health of populations over the life course, and the application of the resulting knowledge to develop and implement policies and actions to improve the health and well-being of the entire community. Actions that result in good health bring greater social, economic, and environmental benefits to the whole population. Such benefits include strengthened social cohesion and citizen engagement, increased national growth and productivity, and improved quality of life. Public health programs have been able to mobilize resources from varied disciplines such as medicine, law, mental health, social services, government, researchers, and practitioners in addressing and preventing elder mistreatment (Ingram, 2003).

Increasingly, elder mistreatment is recognized as a significant public health problem (Public Health Agency of Canada, 2004). Prevention strategies require targeted multidisciplinary approaches and trained professionals with specific knowledge and expertise. Ageism has been identified as a key factor in marginalizing older people and contributing to social isolation and exclusion. The older a person becomes, the greater may be his or her levels of dependency, and thus, the greater the chances of institutionalization as well as the risk of elder mistreatment because of increased vulnerability. Canadian leaders in public health have long been active in developing coordinated community approaches and have established partnership programs, many of which pertain to preventing EA, such as respite care, adult day care, shelters, as well as effective programs for perpetrators.

Due at least in part to Canada's influence, a new paradigm is occurring in many countries, including the rest of North America, shifting the focus from intervention to prevention by placing emphasis on changing the social, behavioral, and environmental factors that contribute to mistreatment (Mercy et al., 1993). This focus furthers an understanding of violence, including the links between physical and psychological violence, the social aspects of the abused and the abusers, the connection among generations, and the risk factors involved for each (Widom, 1998). The intersection of EA and public health continues to evolve as global health is recognized as a rapidly emerging policy field. It behooves all governments to formulate a global health strategy, one that incorporates principles of human rights, a concrete plan of action, a timeline, and identification of achievable and measurable goals.

INFORMATION AND COMMUNICATION TECHNOLOGIES: THE FUTURE OF PREVENTION

Consequences of elder mistreatment for older persons are profound: lifelong ill health, increased hospitalizations, premature institutionalization, premature or even untimely death (Podnieks & Thomas, 2017). In spite of statistics demonstrating the growing magnitude of elder mistreatment worldwide, such mistreatment continues to be underappreciated as a public health problem. Even nowadays, considerably fewer resources are devoted to elder mistreatment than to more recognized public health problems such as child abuse and sexual abuse. The recent Global Status Report on Violence Prevention (2014) calls for a scaling up of violence prevention programs in all countries, including stronger legislation and enhanced services for victims. The report also advocates for better and more effective use of data to inform the development and implementation of prevention programs and to measure effectiveness and progress. Margaret Chan, WHO Director-General, states that the findings "show us that indeed violence is preventable," beginning with an understanding of risk factors and followed by targeted strategies (2014).

Foege et al. (1995) similarly stated that global violence is not inevitable. The idea that violence can be prevented can change the future by promoting the identification of those at risk for mistreatment. Given an understanding of the risks, the public would expect and demand that preventive steps be taken. Social media can be enormously powerful in influencing public opinion, as demonstrated by the abuse scandal involving a prominent football coach and youth at Penn State University, where action was eventually taken (Begin, 2010). With the whole world watching, the message was clear: Violence would not be tolerated. Despite such hopeful occurrences, the implementation of strategies for preventing EA continues to lag behind strategies for preventing other forms of violence.

The recent Global Status Report on Violence Prevention (2014) found that fewer than a third of countries surveyed (26%) reported implementing campaigns aimed at educating professionals to recognize the signs and risk factors of elder mistreatment and to improve their problem-solving and case management skills. Only 23% of these countries claimed to be developing public information or awareness campaigns on elder mistreatment, citing, among other reasons, a lack of technological sophistication. As shown in the summary of practices in addressing EA in six countries (Table 8.1), fostering awareness tends to be the most promising and prevalent activity. Although only a small number of countries have strong awareness programs, the use of technology to quickly and effectively communicate is becoming more widespread and is promoting a worldwide dialogue on violence prevention, changing traditional prevention messaging, and making such messages available to wider audiences (World Health Organization, 2014). Social media are changing the entire landscape of communication. Consequently, the implications for global health are far reaching, unprecedented, and unfathomable.

Social media, which started to attract attention in the early 2000s, have rapidly become the most influential phenomenon of the past decade. Mobile phones and other technological forms of social communication have become central tools for sharing information and ideas among organizations, governments, educational institutions, political entities, nongovernmental organizations (NGOs), and public service and policy groups. In fact, 75% of the world's population, including the developing world, has access to a mobile phone—a number that rises to 90% in Russia and 94% in Iraq (Ranck, 2012). The accelerating rate of adoption of mobile communications and phone applications has profound implications for global health (World Bank, 2012). Although a relatively new area, the use of ICT holds great promise for public health, particularly in preventing, detecting, and treating elder mistreatment (Meurn, 2012). Websites, interactive platforms, blogs, chat rooms, and public service announcements can call attention to the issue. Hotlines and information shared on the Internet are being used effectively to detect and report abuse.

Further proof of the impact of technology is seen in its application to health literacy. Former U.S. Assistant Secretary for Health, Dr. Howard K. Koh made a powerful case for professionals to communicate in plain language, using accurate, easy-to-use information about health issues, thereby enabling people to take action to protect and promote their own health and wellness (Koh, 2012). Basic health literacy is fundamental to putting sound public health guidance into practice and enabling people to follow recommendations. Health literacy is a foundational pillar upon which the information, ideas, and knowledge presented in this chapter rests. There is often a chasm of understanding between what professionals know, and how they communicate what they know, and what patients, consumers, care recipients, and providers know and are able to process and understand. Levels of literacy need to be assessed, and communication needs to be tailored accordingly.

Older adults nowadays have lower average levels of education than younger people, and many are less "literate" in using technology to access information about health issues or to communicate with others. Literacy levels, therefore, must be assessed and respected by all disciplines intervening in EA. Technology offers speedy methods of communication, which lend themselves to short, pithy messages reducing verbiage and forcing the author to get to the point simply. What better example than Twitter with its limit of 140 characters? However, without prompting, many older adults are not likely to use this form of communication.

Recently, there has been an increase in the use of electronic checklists within hospitals for various surgical procedures (Gawande, 2011). These checklists could be adapted to include screening items that would increase the detection rate of elder mistreatment. With tablets and electronic records becoming more available, a unique and unprecedented opportunity exists for healthcare professionals to play a key role in early identification and prevention. Technology can also be used to educate healthcare providers remotely on how to recognize and address elder mistreatment (Meurn, 2012) while respecting the human rights of those who have been abused as well as the abusers.

Professionals may not be the only ones to take advantage of the benefits offered by new technologies. A 2014 Pew Research Centre study, Older Adults and Technology, reported that most seniors in the United States own cell phones and computers. Study results highlight the growing numbers of older adults adopting technologies to communicate, stay connected, and enhance the quality of everyday living. Sensors are tracking movements and activities of older persons, providing safety and supervision effectively and unobtrusively. These devices could also be adapted to become key instruments in prevention and early detection of potentially harmful situations. Other modes of telecommunication that have the potential to impact prevention programs include websites, online training, webinars, and the many uses of mobile phones featuring Short Message Service (SMS). Increased access to technology coupled with the rapid introduction of new, faster, easier technologies provide bountiful opportunities to prevent, detect, and treat EA. SMS has been one form of messaging for educational awareness programs. SMS can be used in tandem with online tools, as it was during the Haiti earthquake and the crisis in Libya (IOM, 2012).

By its very nature, social media can be used to foster an inclusive global health community—a community in which public health leaders demonstrate the powerful potential of technologies to create safe and healthy communities with the help of such platforms as Twitter, Facebook, Google, and other communication "apps" that continue to proliferate. E-mapping and collaborative workspaces, such as Second Life, offer new ways to collaborate, whereas crowd sourcing and crowd funding continue to demonstrate an unparalleled impact to harness ideas and raise money.

TOOLS FOR INTERACTION, SUPPORT, MONITORING, AND COLLABORATION

Gaming is another tool for interaction that allows communications and online interactions among many people at the same time. Sawyer (n.d.) proposes that gaming has the potential to influence behavioral changes through empowerment. For example, a game has been created that engages Kenyan youth in HIV prevention. Organizations have been able to identify, package, and make available accessible tools for people to model and play with health as a form of intervention. A game used to empower women, the AWARE/OWARE game, was adapted from an African game played 7,000 years ago. It is a useful educational and empowerment lesson for social change or "a game for good." The game is designed to explore the challenges and successes in moving toward aspects of female human rights and politics (Art Works for Change, 2015). Many older adults started playing games with their children and are still playing them. Such games, played across generations and by members of diverse groups, can be used to teach about health, inform people about human rights, encourage shared learning, and raise awareness of EA. Even adult coloring books, now widely popular, can be used as a teaching/prevention tool. Games can provide people with frameworks focused on positive health behaviors so that they can make better choices. An important and highly engaging opportunity exists for the development of games that directly address the prevention of EA.

Assistive devices, another type of technological advance, are increasingly marketed and indeed can be helpful, but often are priced beyond the means of the average older adult. Questions arise around the rights of older adults to access assistive devices and products that can enable them to remain healthy and independent and to age in place. Some adults are being "oversold" technology or services in contracts that are legally "unfair" and that border on or constitute financial abuse. Technology is also promoted as an aid to those who care for older adults. Although the occupational health and safety of caregivers needs to be protected, it is important that it not be at the expense of social interaction. Robots, for example, may be able to perform some functions although they are not substitutes for human contact.

Technology has been used to monitor the quality of care provided to older adults in senior care settings. However, devices such as surveillance cameras intrude on older persons' rights to privacy and may also jeopardize the rights of care providers. There is a need to examine the relationship between the desire for helpful new technologies and the legal implications of surveillance as a way of preventing EA or neglect (Gutman, Watts, & Columbo, 2010).

Technologies such as those mentioned above can provide new ways to share resources, solve problems, raise money, engage the public, and collaborate worldwide. They have the potential to democratize access to expertise, resources, and tools, and facilitate building an inclusive global health community while closing the gap between the "have" and "have not" countries. Public health leaders have an unmatched opportunity to lead the way in demonstrating the powerful potential these technologies bring to create safe and healthy communities (Ranck, 2011) while avoiding potential legal and ethical pitfalls. Although there are many exciting innovations inherent in the field of technology and social media, a darker side must also be acknowledged: There is a potential for harm as well as for benefits, possible negative outcomes along with the positive. Even emails, phone calls, and text messages can become conduits for various forms of abuse. Education and precaution are key to preventing harmful activities, such as cyberbullying, loss of privacy and security, scams, data ownership rather than data sharing, and financial abuse.

POLICY BOX

To help older persons become informed technological citizens:

- Help them understand how to use current technologies; ensure they are able to learn how to use new ones

- Ensure that the poor have access to technologies—may require design of new approaches

- Support the development and testing of a curriculum to teach people how to use the new media in the most informed way

- Develop rapid evaluation methodologies to ensure that interventions are evidence-based and successful

WEBSITE FOR WOMEN ENDURING ABUSE: AN INNOVATIVE EXAMPLE OF THE USE OF TECHNOLOGY

A new research project under way in Canada aims to offer women facing violence greater safety by providing practical help, support, and resources. Designed for women in domestic abuse situations, the project has already helped a number of older women, although the majority of the women benefiting from the program so far are younger. The goal is to provide women with confidential, personalized action plans so that they can escape an abusive situation or at least minimize their risk as they decide whether to leave or stay where they are. The process begins with a phone call to the study line. A trained researcher first ensures that the woman calling has a secure email address and a safe place to use a computer, such as a library, a community center, a café, or the home of a trusted friend or family member, and that she knows how to clear her browser and search history. Once she logs onto the website, researchers help assess her risk of harm. Women at risk are provided with resources selected by domestic violence experts, police, and child protection staff. A woman receives a tailored, individualized plan for her own safety. Over the course of a year, each woman will receive four online follow-up sessions to help her deal with the long-term physiological effects of violence, which can include chronic pain, panic attacks, anxiety, and depression. These sessions shift the focus from short-term help in a crisis to long-term support.

Researchers are exploring whether the website can help victims who are reluctant to use women's shelters. Fewer than one in five Canadian women overall access support from violence services, so an online service could be an important alternative. A similar study (Campbell, Webster, & Glass, 2009) in the United States found that a computerized program helped women take steps to increase their safety. The women reported that the interventions made them feel supported while protecting their privacy.

According to the Young Women's Christian Association (YWCA), a woman will leave an abusive relationship on average seven times before she leaves for good; an older woman may never leave. A hope for the Canadian project is that women will be able to monitor their own safety and have an escape plan in place (Corpuz-Bosshart, 2015). The plan can include practical and effective tasks such as keeping bank accounts, passports, and other identification in a safe place. The website project is not just a safety plan but also a plan to build confidence. The more access women have to resources, the more powerful they become. Although most women in the research project are not yet elderly, this research clearly has implications for older women, given that EA is often domestic abuse grown old.

CALL FOR RESEARCH AND EVALUATION

The health sector, including public health, has been slow to adopt new technologies to advance their agendas. There is a need for research in this area to better understand the issues and to determine how these technologies can be coupled with rigorous and ongoing evaluation to ensure their efficiency and effectiveness. A powerful role exists for technologies to help countries to collaborate, share resources, and work toward developing effective, efficient, and responsive service delivery systems building on the successes of their global partners. Programs and projects from other fields and disciplines will further reinforce the power of new technologies to build community capacity, professional competencies, and public engagement and confidence in the field of EA.

Further discussion concerning the interface between EA and public health should focus on how new technologies can help diminish the "digital divide" among generations. The current generation of subject matter experts is embracing and transferring knowledge and skills to the next generation, whose primary mode of communication and method of work is through the use of ICT, including collaborative platforms. Meurn (2012) offers recommendations on ways for global health communities to harness the power of technology to advance the prevention and treatment of EA worldwide. These include full-landscape analysis of the intersection between ICT and the field of violence prevention, with particular emphasis on the mobile phone in relation to the developing world, as well as the following measures:

- Learning from other fields using new platforms for information sharing and collaboration and sharing data and lessons learned

- Developing common metrics for monitoring and evaluation

- Exploring issues concerning user privacy, data sharing and reporting

- Examining the factors leading to the instigation and continued perpetration of violence, such as poverty, lack of access to healthcare, lack of access to education, and economic inequality, which can set the stage for abusive behavior

A public health approach measures and analyzes the full range of factors and determinants known to influence and contribute to health. Evidence from research and other sources link key health issues to their determinants and show how these factors combine to cause health or illness. Such issues can be addressed in collaboration with community public health workers using computers and mobile phones to help expand access to healthcare and education.

Although communication is vitally important for transmitting information to help both professionals and the public in recognizing and preventing EA and treating those who have been abused as well as the abusers, a solid research foundation must first lay the groundwork for such communications. To that end, the public health model shown in Figure 8.1 provides an essential framework for testing and evaluating the impacts of strategies for preventing abuse and the effectiveness of treatment options. Research on risk factors, taking into account the importance of characteristics and situations that can either singly or in combination foster neglect or abuse, will make it easier to identify those persons who are most vulnerable to abuse. The public health model is intended to be dynamic and applicable to succeeding generations of older people. Consideration must also be given to the idea that each generation may respond differently to diverse and evolving methods of communication such as traditional media, the Internet, and social networks, and to treatments and prevention strategies.

RESEARCH BOX

- To what extent are the following questions researchable, and if they are, how should we design studies to tackle them?

- What are the most effective modes of communication for impressing young people about the importance of recognizing and preventing EA?

- To what extent are there cultural and ethnic differences across populations of the world in addressing EA?

- Why are some societies actively attacking EA issues while others are not?

- Are risk factors for EA similar across cultures? If not, what are the differences and why do they exist?

(continued)

- Is there a best practices approach to developing legislation to combat EA?

- What is the best way to train healthcare providers to respect older adults and to provide support and assistance in cases of abuse?

- Which types of prevention strategies are the most successful?

SUMMARY

This chapter has examined the conditions and interactions that can ultimately lead to the prevention of EA, within a public health framework and compatible with human rights. The ideas presented here are intended to foster a richness of imagination and lead to new directions in applied research. We have presented a public health model that focuses first on public awareness. We stress that it is important to go beyond promotion of public awareness of EA, now a worldwide phenomenon with some degree of success. Events held annually for WEAAD may fostered continuing worldwide improvements in methods of detection, intervention, treatment, and ultimately prevention, as illustrated in the public health model of EA. The elements of this model need to be tested, and the best approaches to each of its elements need to be developed. Furthermore, a better understanding of the connections among the various elements of the model is needed.

In this chapter, we described current initiatives, policies, and progress in six countries across the globe. The importance of public health leadership in the prevention and response to EA must be stressed. Although resources are limited, public health agencies as well as other agencies have a wealth of data, insights, and dedication developed through experience and research. They are supported in their work by dedicated staff from NGOs.

This chapter also explored the new world of information and communications technologies as tools for cooperation. The public health field will benefit from applying technologies creatively to enhance awareness and prevention (Ranck, 2011). The buzzword "technological citizen" refers to understanding how to use current technologies and continuing to relearn them as the new tools constantly evolve. We noted that there is a need for an evidence base concerning the effectiveness of new technologies for EA prevention. We recognize that the theoretical foundations of a field describe and inform practice and provide the primary means to guide future developments. We suggest that these ideas can influence practices and research and lead to new knowledge and alternatives for preventing EA (Podnieks & Thomas, 2017). We highlight a global public health phenomenon that has received worldwide attention, one that promotes the concept that all individuals have a social responsibility to take action against EA.

Thought-Provoking Questions

1. How might a better understanding of EA help in the design of policies and programs?

2. Which types of training programs might be valuable for public health workers in relation to the potential cases of EA they might encounter?

3. What are some important risk factors for EA and how might they be neutralized?

4. Why is a human rights perspective important for EA?

5. Why is it important to develop a dynamic, rather than static, model of public health and EA?

6. How can advances in technology benefit elders who might be subject to abuse?

REFERENCES

Acierno, R., Hernandez, M. A., Amstadter, A. B., Resnick, H. S., Steve, K., Muzzy, W., & Kilpatrick, D. G. (2010). Prevalence and correlates of emotional, physical, sexual, and financial abuse and potential neglect in the United States: The National Elder Mistreatment Study. *American Journal of Public Health, 100,* 292–297. doi:10.2105/AJPH.2009.163089

AWARE/OWARE—Art Works for Change. (2015, January 15). Retrieved from http://www.artworksforchange.org

Begin, M. (2010). *Social determinants of health: The Canadian facts.* J. Mikkonen & D. Raphael (Eds.). Toronto, Canada: York University School of Health and Management.

Bonnie, R. J., & Wallace, R. B. (Eds.). (2003). *Elder mistreatment: Abuse, neglect, and exploitation in an aging America.* Washington, DC: National Academies Press.

Campbell, J. C., Webster, D. W., & Glass, N. (2009). The danger assessment: Validation of a lethality risk assessment instrument for intimate partner femicide. *Journal of Interpersonal Violence, 24*, 653–674. doi:10.1177/0886260508317180

Canadian Network for the Prevention of Elder Abuse. (2017). New Quebec government action plan to counter elder mistreatment (2017–2022) - "Québec keeps innovating". Retrieved from https://cnpea.ca/en/about-cnpea/blog/745-new-quebec-government-action-plan-to-counter-elder-mistreatment-2017-2022-québec-keeps-innovating

Columbia University Mailman School of Public Health. (2009). The relationship of human rights to health (Human Rights Learning Module). Retrieved from http://www.columbia.edu/itc/hs/pubhealth/modules/humanRights/relationship.html

Comijs, H. C., Pot, A. M., Smit, J. H., Bouter, L. M., & Jonker, C. (1998). Elder abuse in the community: Prevalence and consequences. *Journal of the American Geriatrics Society, 46*, 885–888. doi: 10.1111/j.1532-5415.1998.tb02724.x

Cook-Daniels, L. (1997). Lesbian, gay male, bisexual, and transgendered elders: Elder abuse and neglect issues. *Journal of Elder Abuse & Neglect, 9*(2), 35–49. doi:10.1300/J084v09n02_04

Cooke, J. G. (2009). *Public health in Africa: A report of the CSIS Global Health Policy Center.* Washington, DC: Center for Strategic and International Studies. Retrieved from https://csis-prod.s3.amazonaws.com/s3fs-public/legacy_files/files/media/csis/pubs/090420_cooke_pubhealthafrica_web.pdf

Cooper, C., Selwood, A., & Livingston, G. (2008). The prevalence of elder abuse and neglect: A systematic review. *Age and Ageing, 37*(2), 151–160. doi:10.1093/ageing/afm194

Corpuz-Bosshart, L. (2015, February 17). New online support tool for victims of partner violence. *University of British Columbia News.* Retrieved from https://news.ubc.ca/2015/02/17/new-online-support-tool-for-victims-of-partner-violence

Cruz, A. D. (2014, January 23). Elder Abuse & LGBT older adults: Recent news & research [Blog post]. Retrieved from https://nyceac.org/elder-justice-dispatch-elder-abuse-lgbt-older-adults-recent-news-research

Ferreira, M. (2008). Elder abuse in Africa: what policy and legal provisions are there to address the violence? *Journal of Elder Abuse and Neglect, 16*(2), 17–32. doi: 10.1300/j084v16no2_02.

Flynn, D. (2005). What's wrong with rights? Rethinking human rights and responsibilities. *Australian Social Work, 58*(3), 244–256. doi:10.1111/j.1447-0748.2005.00218.x

Foege, W. H., Rosenberg, M. L., & Mercy, J. A.(1995). Public health and violence prevention. *Current Issues in Public Health, 1*, 2–9.

Fredvang, M., & Biggs, S. (2012, August). *The rights of older persons: Protections and gaps under human rights law.* Social Policy Working Paper No. 16. Melbourne,

Australia: Brotherhood of St. Laurence and University of Melbourne Centre for Public Policy. Retrieved from https://social.un.org/ageing-working-group/documents/fourth/Rightsofolderpersons.pdf

Gawande, A. (2011). *The checklist manifesto: How to get things right*. New York, NY: Picador.

Georgantzi, N. (2012). *Elder abuse and neglect in the European Union.* Paper presented at the third working session of the U.N. Open-ended Working Group on Ageing. August 21–24, New York, NY. Retrieved from https://social.un.org/ageing-working-group/documents/ElderAbuseNGOEWG2012.pdf

Gutman, G., Watts, L., & Colombo, M. (2010). ISG*INPEA round table: Gerontechnology as an elder abuse issue. *Gerontechnology, 9*(2), 344. doi:10.4017/gt.2010.09.02.299.00

Harrison, J., & Riggs, D. W. (Eds.). (2006). Editorial: LGBT ageing. *Gay & Lesbian Issues and Psychology Review, 2*, 42–43. Retrieved from: https://groups.psychology.org.au/Assets/Files/GLIP_Review_Vol2_No2.pdf

Iborra, I., Garcia, Y., & Grau, E. (2013). Spain: Public health and elder mistreatment in Spain. In A. Phelan (Ed.), *International perspectives in elder abuse* (pp. 168–187). London, UK: Routledge.

Ingram, E. M. (2003). Expert panel recommendations on elder mistreatment using a public health framework. *Journal of Elder Abuse & Neglect, 15*(2), 45–65. doi:10.1300/J084v15n02_03

Koh, H. & Osborne, D. (2012, May 8). *Dr. Howard Koh, assistant secretary for HHS, talks about boosting health literacy to move beyond the cycle of costly crisis care* [Podcast HLOL #77, transcript]. Natick, MA: Health Literacy Consulting. Retrieved from https://healthliteracy.com/2012/05/08/dr-howard-k-koh-assistant-secretary-for-hhs-talks-about-boosting-health-literacy-to-move-beyond-the-cycle-of-costly-crisis-care-hlol-77/

Lachs, M. S., Williams, C., O'Brien, S., Hurst, L., & Horwitz, R. (1997). Risk factors for reported elder abuse and neglect: A nine-year observational cohort study. *Gerontologist, 37*, 469–474. doi:10.1093/geront/37.4.469

Lindert, J., de Luna, J., Torres-Gonzales, F., Barros, H. & Ioannidi-Kopolou, E. (2013). Abuse and neglect of older persons in seven cities in seven countries in Europe: a cross-sectional community study. *International Journal of Public Health, 58*, 121–132. doi: 10:1007/s00038-012-0388-3.

Lorman, J. (2015). *Czech Republic: Zivot 90, elder mistreatment in the Czech Republic.* Unpublished document.

Macfarlane, S., Raceles, M., & Muli-Muslime, F. (2000, September 2). Public health in developing countries. *The Lancet, 356*, 841–846.

Magar, S. T., & Gurung, A. (2015). Year book of senior citizens 2016. Battisputali, Kathmandu, Nepal: Ageing Nepal. Retrieved from http://ageingnepal.org/wp-content/uploads/2016/02/Final-year-book-2016.pdf

Mann, J. M., Goslin, L., Gruskin, S., Brennan, T., Lazzarini, Z., & Fineberg, H. V. (1994). Health and human rights. *Health and Human Rights, 1*(1), 6–23.

Marsh, J. C. (2003). The Social work response to violence. *Social Work, 48,* 437– 438.

Mercy, J. A., Butchart, A., Rosenberg, M. L., Dahlberg, A., & Harvey, A. (2008). Preventing violence in developing countries: A framework for action. *International Journal of Injury Control and Safety Promotion, 15*(4), 197–208. doi:10.1080/17457300802406955

Mercy, J. A., Rosenberg, M. L., Powell, K. E., Broome, C. V., & Roper, W. L. (1993). Public health policy for preventing violence. *Health Affairs, 12,* 7–29.

Meurn, C. (2012). Foundations of mPreventViolence: Integrating violence prevention and information and communications technologies. In Institute of Medicine & National Research Council, *Communication and technology for violenc prevention: Workshop summary* (pp. 43–86). and Washington, DC: National Academies Press. Retrieved from https://www.nap.edu/read/13352/chapter/9.

O'Lougham, A. & Duggan, J. (1998). *Abuse, neglect and mistreatment of older people: an exploratory study* (Report No. 52). Dublin, Ireland: National Council on Ageing and Older People. Retrieved from http://hdl.handle.net/10147/44465

Perel-Levin, S. (2008). *Discussing screening for elder abuse at primary health care level.* Geneva, Switzerland: World Health Organization. Retrieved from http://www.who.int/ageing/publications/Discussing_Elder_Abuseweb.pdf

Pillemer, K. & Finkelhor, D. (1988). Prevalence of elder abuse: A random sample survey. *Gerontologist, 28*(1), 51–57.

Ploeg, J., Lohfeld, L., & Walsh, C. A. (2013). What is "elder abuse"? Voices from the margin: The views of underrepresented Canadian older adults. *Journal of Elder Abuse & Neglect, 25,* 396–424. doi:10.1080/08946566.2013.780956

Podnieks, E., & Thomas, C. (2017). The consequences of elder abuse and neglect. In X. Q. Dong (Ed.), *Elder abuse: Research, practice and policy* (pp.109-123). New York, NY: Springer International.

Ranck, J. (2011). *Health information and health care: The role of technology in unlocking data and wellness: A discussion paper.* Washington, DC: United Nations Foundation & Vodafone Foundation Technology Partnership.

Ranck, J. (2012). *Information and communications technologies and the future of global health.* IOM Forum on Global Violence Prevention.

SAGE. (2015). Services and advocacy for LGBT elders (2012-2018). Retrieved from http://sageusa.org

Sawyer B. (n.d.). Ben Sawyer on Games for Health—MIT Media Lab. Retrieved from https://www.media.mit.edu

Sedlak, A. J. (1991). *National incidence and prevalence of child abuse and neglect: 1988* (Revised report). Rockville, MD: Westat.

Tenenbaum, D. (2012, May 4). Study finds high rate of victimization among gays, lesbians and bisexuals. University of Wisconsin-Madison News.

Thomas, C. (2000). The first national study of elder abuse and neglect: Contrast with results from other studies. *Journal of Elder Abuse & Neglect, 12*(1), 1–14. doi:10.1300/J084v12n01_01

Thomas, C., Tatara, T., Gertig, J., Kuzmeskus, L. B., Jay, K., Duckhorn, E., ... Croos, J. (1998). *The National Elder Abuse Incidence Study, final report*. Washington, DC: Administration for Children and Families and Administration on Aging, U.S. Department of Health and Human Services. Retrieved from https://secure .ce-credit.com/articles/100860/ElderAbuseIncidentReport.pdf

United Nations General Assembly. (1948). *Universal Declaration of Human Rights*. Retrieved from http://www.ohchr.org/EN/UDHR/Pages/UDHRIndex.aspx

Widom, C. S. (1998). Child victims: searching for opportunities to break the cycle of violence. *Applied and Preventive Psychology, 7*, 225–234.

World Bank. (2012). Mobile phone access reaches three quarters of world population. Retrieved from http://www.worldbank.org/en/news/press-release/2012/07/17/ mobile-phone-access-reaches-three-quarters-planets-population

World Health Organization. (1998). *Health Promotion Glossary*. (WHO/HPR/ HEP/98.1). Geneva, Switzerland: Author. Retrieved from http://www.who.int/ healthpromotion/about/HPR%20Glossary%201998.pdf

World Health Organization. (2014). *Global status report on violence prevention 2014*. Geneva, Switzerland: Author. Retrieved from http://www.who.int/violence_ injury_prevention/violence/status_report/2014/report/report/en

World Health Organization, & The International Network for the Prevention of Elder Abuse. (2002). *Missing voices: Views of older persons on elder abuse: A study of eight countries*. Geneva, Switzerland: Authors. Retrieved from http://apps.who .int/iris/bitstream/10665/67371/1/WHO_NMH_VIP_02.1.pdf

9

SUMMATIONS AND CONCLUDING THOUGHTS
Pamela B. Teaster and Jeffrey E. Hall

It is our intent in this concluding chapter to summarize the major points regarding elder abuse (EA) presented in the preceding chapters. We conclude the chapter by taking one last opportunity to encourage exploration and initiation of system-level efforts to solve a major public health problem.

PERSPECTIVES AND POSITIONS ON EA: A SUMMATION

Throughout the book, we have attempted to present a cogent argument, made in a variety of ways and by a diverse array of scholars, that EA is a public health problem, that EA is public health's problem, and that EA is the public's health problem. First, EA is a genuine public health problem. A growing and reputable body of scholarship has been amassed since the 1960s as testament to the fact that no longer is the problem an individualized one or relegated to the status of "simply a family matter" as it was once purported to be (Acierno et al., 2010; Lachs, Williams, O'Brien, Pillemer, & Charlson, 1998; Laumann, Leitsch, & Waite, 2008; Teaster et al., 2006). Rather, said first and most eloquently by the late Robert Butler (2008), an overarching reason that EA occurs is its insidious roots in

---

Disclaimer: The findings and conclusions in this chapter are those of the authors and do not necessarily represent the official position of the Centers for Disease Control and Prevention.

the problem of ageism, a problem that has yet to make its way into public consciousness or the public lexicon.

Unlike the "isms" of sexism and racism, ageism is barely acknowledged as existing or as an oppressive or discriminatory problem that affects over a third of the population. The reach of this "ism" is especially damaging, as recognized by the Age Discrimination in Employment Act of 1967, which covers all those at 40 years of age and above Moreover, former Surgeon General Jocelyn Elders recognized that "we all have got to come to grips with our isms" (Kate's Bookshelf, 2014). We believe that the time has come to confront the dangers of ageism and its implications for all our shared health and well-being.

Second, as we did in Chapter 1, we stress that EA is public health's problem. It is public health's problem because EA is a form of preventable violence, and prevention efforts to assuage the problem fit squarely within the wheelhouse of public health vis-à-vis primary, secondary, and tertiary preventive measures. Furthermore, attempts to understand the scope of EA are analogous to the current epidemiologic surveillance efforts related to forms of interpersonal violence such as intimate partner violence (IPV), sexual violence, and child abuse. Information derived from these surveillance efforts has provided critical insights and lessons have been learned regarding the considerations, methods, and approaches required to accurately measure and monitor the prevalence and incidence of abusive, neglectful, or exploitive behaviors.

In addition, EA is public health's problem because public health routinely brings together diverse disciplines and diverse actors at local, state, and national levels to confront public problems impacting the public's health and is able to quantify the eradication or reduction of the public health problem. Recent and analogous infectious disease–based examples are efforts related to Ebola, HIV/AIDS, human papillomavirus (HPV), swine flu, Zika, H1N1, and obesity (United Nations General Assembly, 2016). More distant but ongoing efforts of the public health community are those related to cancer, smoking cessation, and motor vehicle accidents. We are learning that a one-size-fits-all solution to these problems may not prove fruitful as our field grows from infancy to one that is more mature and sophisticated—that is, what works for a younger population may not work for an older one. Complex problems require broader engagement and involvement of relevant parties inside and outside public health to ensure that the devised age-cognizant solutions stand the best chance of achieving relevance and success.

EA is public health's problem because it stands in direct opposition to the goal of public health to promote healthy aging, because abuse is the antithesis of a state of health. EA can be both a contributor and a promoter of both chronic and acute diseases as well as early death (Choi & Mayer, 2000). Conversely, chronic and acute diseases can easily contribute to vulnerabilities to EA (Namkee et al., 2000). The consequences of both of these scenarios have implications for multiple sectors of the workforce, including but not limited to medicine, social work, law, and business. The health effects can be even more pernicious, because the consequences of EA can affect the health and well-being of present and future generations in terms of the transmission of violence (Mercy, Rosenberg, Powell, Broome, & Roper, 1993), economic stressors, and health stressors, not to mention conflicts within families that may persist for decades.

We propose that public health offers viable and tested frameworks for comprehensively addressing the problem at micro levels through macro levels, thus offering the potential to effect real population health change at the level of the individual as well as at the level of policy and ideology. The chapters of the book represent specific ways in which public health intersects with these spheres.

In Chapter 2, Irving and Hall explained how the issue of EA is both a public health problem and a human rights violation (Ingram, 2003). They suggest that the mission and tools of public health complement sectors in society already involved in intervention and prevention efforts. By presenting EA as a preventable and remediable public health problem, they are able to embed EA within the core functions of public health (i.e., assessment, policy development, and assurance) and the 10 essential public health services. These services were developed by a work group operating under the auspices of the Centers for Disease Control and Prevention's Public Health Practice Program Office and the Office of Disease Prevention and Health Promotion to explain public health, clarify its role within a larger healthcare system, and provide accountability by linking public health performance to health outcomes. Irving and Hall describe ways that public health can address EA using each of the services as touchstones for public health work but caution that leveraging "public health's inherent talents and native ways of serving the population generally and older adults specifically" can be accomplished only through the commitment of adequate and dedicated human and social capital.

Continuing with the theme of the core functions, Jadhav and Holsinger (Chapter 3) explored the intersection of EA in public health law and health services administration by using specific examples from the Commonwealth of Kentucky via a lens of purposeful living. The authors stress that understanding the health consequences of an act of abuse is critical to establishing a public health interface. They suggest that the WHO definition of public health is perhaps the most applicable, as it includes prolonging life and promoting health. In addition, public health administration has as its purview implementing laws that keep older adults safe in long-term care facilities as well as reducing health disparities among older adults. The authors strengthen the association between public health administration and EA by proposing a framework derived from the core functions of public health: prevalence, diagnosis, societal impact, and preventability (PDSP).

Chapter 4, by Ramsey-Klawsnik, begins a second section of the book, in which we consider special populations in relation to public health and the issue of EA. Although IPV is typically regarded as an issue involving younger adults, the problem as it affects older adults is often disregarded. Ramsey-Klawsnik's chapter is organized around allegations of IPV with which the author is familiar and that were reported to Adult Protective Services (APS). The cases proffered are vehicles to highlight the dynamics of the situation and to elucidate how these cases are associated with public health. Ramsey-Klawsnik points to the important education function that public health professionals can perform to help victims understand their rights and available interventions, which is especially important because domestic violence often increases in consequences and severity as individuals age. IPV experienced in late life resembles the abuse that younger, battered women encounter; however, IPV encountered by older women can also occur in the provision of care for chronic conditions. Inappropriate interventions to stop it can result in greater harm to the victim. Public health professionals and academics stand ready to help the public understand social justice issues related to IPV of older adults—including the notion that such violence should not be an exception granted or ignored under the special treatment given to spousal relationships, but rather a criminal offense requiring appropriate, formal action, regardless of the sex of the perpetrator. Ramsey-Klawsnik opines that public health professionals are in an excellent position to assist older adults in situations involving IPV, particularly in regard to social messaging and intervention.

The consideration of EA in special populations continues in Chapter 5 with Cox and Jervis's discussion of EA and American Indians. Cox and Jervis note that advances on the topic are being made because tribes are becoming increasingly aware of the problem. The authors are quick to point out that the problem is a nascent one for Native populations, but that the problem was noted in the scholarly literature as problematic even in the 1980s. During that decade, Brown (1989) used a sample of 110 Navajo elders and their families and reported that 16% disclosed being physically abused. Sudden-onset dependency, mental health issues for elders and caregivers, and neglect because of caregiver weariness or economic hardship were often associated with these events (Brown, 1989). Cox and Jervis point out that colonialism disrupted and supplanted the lifeways of Native American elders and older adults, who had traditionally been the repository of wealth as well as cultural, spiritual, and moral resources for their tribes. Such disruptions resulted in the devaluation of elders, placing them in positions of vulnerability and dependency, and situated them as victims of spiritual abuse (i.e., intentionally tearing down belief systems). As early as the 1970s, Baker (1975), Butler (1975), and Burston (1975) stressed that EA should understood as a public health issue needing structural as well as community- and individual-level solutions, a perspective especially critical to Native communities. The authors stress that fewer than 10% of the 566 federally recognized tribes and Alaskan villages have EA codes in their current tribal codes (Bureau of Indian Affairs, 2014; National Indigenous Elder Justice Initiative, 2014), a problem confounding the increasing number of EA cases coming to tribal attention.

In Chapter 5, Cox and Jervis suggest that public health has a number of roles to play with Native populations. First, public health professionals bring years of expertise understanding and working with Native populations, particularly concerning maternal and child health. Application of ways of working with Native elders and their families on these issues can be exemplars for professionals addressing EA. Second, public health professionals already possess a deep understanding of how to work with communities to prevent and intervene in public health problems such as EA and can apply this understanding to improve caregiving outcomes as well as prevent exploitation of Native elders' resources. Public health officials are also experts in social messaging and public awareness campaigns, and EA campaigns, such as capitalizing on the public attention already given to World Elder Abuse Awareness Day (June 15), is an excellent example of how local public health departments might take action (see Chapter 7).

In Chapter 6, Anetzberger continues our section on special populations and topics by examining the confluence of approaches of nontraditional partners and the public health response to EA. Anetzberger contends that public health can be an important leader in the effort to reduce and eradicate EA, but only if it extends beyond its traditional interface with healthcare. She delineates seven distinct considerations for EA: as a social problem, medical (geriatric) syndrome, aspect of family (domestic) violence, aging (Aging Network) issue, crime, violation of human rights, and public health concern. She notes that these considerations differ according to perception, disciplinary perspective, and primacy of services or programs. In highlighting the problem as one embraced by public health, she holds that a paper presented in 1979 by Hickey and Douglass at the 107th Annual Meeting of the American Public Health Association (later published in 1981) may well have been the inception of the association of the problem with public health.

The paper by Hickey and Douglass reported their research on EA as seen by service-providing professionals and their interface with older adults in community settings. These authors argued that EA was a public health problem, with social workers and public health nurses being most familiar with the problem. Similarly, a decade later, the then Secretary of Health and Human Services, Louis Sullivan, pronounced that EA is a component of family violence and as such is a public health and justice problem. In reviewing public health department websites in 2014, it appeared that little attention to the issue was being given by state public health departments, something Anetzberger remarks is "distressing and a missed opportunity". This is particularly troubling given recognition of the issue as a public health problem by the Second World Assembly on Ageing, which took place in Madrid from April 8 to 12, 2002, and at the National Policy Summit on Elder Abuse, where experts and visionaries came together in Washington, D.C., in December 2001 to develop the first-ever national EA action agenda.

As a remedy, Anetzberger stresses that public health must reach out to partners other than healthcare and proposes that one niche for public health is to align with APS in the arena of public education, suggesting that a public health educational campaign similar to those used with smoking and drunk driving be developed. Another proposed area of public health partnership is with domestic violence and sexual assault programs, particularly in screening for EA. A nexus of public health with the aging network can be found within the area of education and public policy. The intersections of public health, APS, and law enforcement are with the surveillance function of each sector, including the collection, analysis, and dissemination of information. Navarro, Wilber, Yonashiro, and Homeier (2010) have explained that the EA forensic center model was first developed at the University of California in 2003, and launched in January 2006 as the second EA forensic center in the nation, the purpose of which is "to improve the quality of life for vulnerable older and dependent adults who have been victims of abuse and neglect in Los Angeles County." Public health is familiar with how to work in multidisciplinary, interdisciplinary, and transdisciplinary venues. Despite the paucity of outcome studies to illustrate the benefits of multidisciplinary teams/approaches, it is this intersection that Anetzberger suggests holds the most promise for public health to address EA, given how comprehensively the problem can be addressed and that public health has already used this approach successfully in other prevention and intervention campaigns.

Chapter 7 presents an array of prominent programs and campaigns that are addressing EA. Specifically, but by no means exhaustively, the chapter discusses major federal initiatives, national organizations, national entities, and initiatives and campaigns as well as efforts conducted at the individual level. Information presented in the chapter illustrates how the actions of federal and nonfederal agencies and entities are helping elevate and address the problem of EA. Still, the work done thus far emphasizes that more effective communication strategies are critical for primary prevention efforts relating to awareness of and education regarding EA. The chapter highlights the exponential growth and promise of social media, which allows awareness about the issue to be cultivated broadly, continuously, and at reduced costs as compared to paper publications or in-person conferences for a select few. Recently developed and acutely effective venues, such as websites and webinars, have been used to highlight the reality that EA is a public health issue with important, interdisciplinary contributions to address the problem. Limited resources for EA prevention are a persistent drawback to this public health problem. Nevertheless, we are confident that pockets of intervention around the country will continue to strengthen and expand, increasingly emphasizing that EA is not only a national but an international concern, as Chapter 8 by Podnieks and Thomas attests.

Chapter 8 widens the issue of EA beyond the borders of the United States to the international stage. Podnieks and Thomas remind us that population aging represents both a triumph and a failure of public health initiatives. Around the world, an unprecedented number of people are living to older ages, but their vital contributions are too often ignored, and too many experience EA. Framing the problem of EA as one of public health and human rights, the authors stress that public health has a unique stake in the issue because of its goal to alleviate human suffering and promote health and well-being. They emphasize that, as described by Mann et al. (1994), individuals are empowered to lead healthier lives if their needs are met: Consequently and collectively, the public's overall health is improved (Mann et al., 1994). Also, according to Perel-Levin (2008), rather than being paternalistic, this human rights perspective engenders a culture of inclusion and acknowledges and celebrates the uniqueness of each person through an approach that incorporates both individual and global perspectives to resource allocation.

Podnieks and Thomas make suggestions about how to implement human rights practices by providing examples of the inequitable treatment of older lesbian, gay, bisexual, transgender, and questioning (LGBTQ) residents in long-term care facilities (Podnieks & Thomas, 2016). They stress that the World Health Organization (WHO) has disseminated public health concepts that have achieved universal and international recognition, though not all are accompanied by principles of human rights. To address EA through a human rights lens, the authors suggest that a public health model must incorporate elements and explanatory factors hypothesized in other models (e.g., risk factors that facilitate abuse, characteristics of the older person, attributes of the environment, presence of family members with mental illness or substance abuse problems; Lachs, Williams, O'Brien, Hurst, & Horwitz, 1998). Moreover, Podnieks and Thomas assert that EA can be appropriately incorporated in a public health framework to create tools for policy development that can be applied universally.

As a working example of the intersection of public health with EA prevention, Podnieks and Thomas suggest that the Canadian model of population health enjoys a tradition of nationally collaborating programs in public health, community health, and health promotion. The Canadian approach to public health recognizes that interrelated factors and conditions (the social determinants of health) contribute to overall health and that EA is a significant public health problem (Public Health Agency of Canada, 2012). Canadian public health leaders have long been active in developing coordinated community approaches and have established partnership programs pertaining to EA prevention. Moreover, the Canadian approach is being replicated in other countries, notably in the United States, because of its focus on prevention and social, behavioral, and environmental contributors to the problem (Mercy et al., 1993).

These authors add to our earlier emphasis that social media represent a powerful avenue for prevention and emphasize that a meaningful tool for the prevention of EA for global health communities is the power of technology. Public health has already embraced the importance of technology in both primary and secondary prevention efforts. Podnieks and Thomas also explore the new world of information and communications technologies as tools for cooperation. Stressing that the field of public health field must not fall behind in applying technologies creatively, the authors posit that public health must empower "technological citizens"—persons living free from EA.

CONCLUSION

In this book, we have amassed a cadre of highly respected authors, some who were grounded in public health but not EA, and some whose scholarly lives have been dedicated to the problem of EA but with little intersection with public health. Either stance is not surprising, given that, as many of the authors point out, public health is a relative latecomer to the issue of EA (see Anetzberger, Chapter 6). Certainly, in many instances, EA is a preventable problem—one that may well be *the* public health problem of future decades, as well as more obviously public health's problem because this sector does not fully embrace the issue at present. We, the editors, again wish to stress that the time has come for the field of public health to fully embrace the issue of EA, just as it has embraced other, similar prevention efforts. Indeed, older adults are the target population for many public health efforts focused on promoting population health broadly and reducing chronic diseases and their health impacts. Because many diseases and conditions only fully manifest themselves in old age, this period of life may well be a time when significant age-related health inequities become apparent in the United States and internationally. Addressing the socially structured dimensions of life that introduce risks for EA victimization requires commitments extending beyond the few small groups of individuals interested in using public health knowledge to protect older adults. Structural issues require solutions that originate from and are advanced by the macro-level systems that serve entire populations.

We find that, throughout the book, various themes have resonated in the chapters and are a clarion call to public health action. First, the problem of EA is one that has been socially constructed without a solid foundation of public awareness or commitment to intervention or prevention. The problem is left undertreated, under-reported, and under-recognized both in the general public and in public health in particular. We submit that the root of the problem, as cited over 40 years ago by Butler (2008), lies in covert and overt ageism—a problem ripe to be eradicated through the prodigious strengths of public health and the diverse pathways of influence available to the numerous organizations that deliver public health services. These strengths and pathways have already been successfully marshaled and deployed to increase awareness of, and concerted worldwide actions to resolve, public health problems such as smoking, sexually transmitted diseases, childhood diseases, and some other forms of violence.

A second theme is that EA is a problem that demands a number of actors, organizations, and agencies to work together. Public health has historically been a major player in devising and implementing collaborative approaches to population health. Moreover, public health has long been a leader in applying collaborative, multilevel approaches to population health problems, drawing upon everything from bench science to broad public policy initiatives. One highly promising framework that could be adapted and expanded to address EA more broadly is community-based participatory research (CBPR). CBPR is a powerful and insightful method for researching and resolving problems that has been applied successfully in public health to deal with problems such as childhood obesity and domestic violence (Holkup, Tripp-Reimer, Salois, & Weinert, 2004). We challenge professionals, organizations, and alliances working within public health at various levels integrate this and similar population-driven, engagement-centered approaches into multicomponent strategies developed to tackle the problem of EA.

Finally, the socioecological framework for violence prevention utilized within domestic and global public health work is applicable and extendable to EA. Because this model incorporates factors, pathways of influence, and psychosocial process at micro and macro levels of interaction, we know that its use will provide invaluable contributions toward efforts to more effectively prevent the occurrence and reduce the prevalence of this problem. Approaches based on the socioecological model have already been used in research, at least in part, by a small selection of scholars addressing the problem of EA (Roberto & Teaster, 2017; Schiamberg et al., 2011; Teaster, Dugar, & Roberto, 2006). We suggest that future research, policy, and practice efforts incorporate this model, particularly as it attempts to analyze, understand, and approach the complexities of EA such as polyvictimization (Ramsey-Klawsnik & Heisler, 2014) and the characteristics of family and community systems and dynamics associated with EA perpetration and victimization uniquely and jointly. Heeding this advice may be particularly critical when developing new environmental or policy-based actions or instruments or evaluating the capability of existing actions or instruments to reach and effectively prevent EA in the diverse local settings where it may occur. Such a model may prove useful in identifying the many different intervening variables and pathways of influence that must be altered or accounted for to achieve desired prevention outcomes locally, nationally, or internationally.

We recognize that the ability of public health to address these problems is enormously promising, *if* public health builds infrastructures and formally commits to the systematic education of its workforce and partnership networks on the topic of EA and techniques for its prevention. To be sure, public health has already invested resources to address the issue—notably, in the form of the uniform definitions and recommended core data elements for use in EA surveillance that were promulgated in 2016. However, we stress that there is so much more that is right and timely for public health to embrace, and so many more ways that the social capital of the public health field can be strategically leveraged for good effect on behalf of older adults.

Throughout this book, we have argued that EA is a public health problem and that EA may well be among the most under-recognized and under-resourced population health problems of the early 21st century. Public health has frameworks, tools, approaches, relationships, structures, systems, and a variety of agents and organizations poised to address the problem of EA. The imprimatur of the growing population of older adults and the character of demographic transitions occurring globally provide the perfect rationale for action—now.

REFERENCES

Acierno, R., Hernandez, M. A., Amstadter, A. B., Resnick, H. S., Steve, K., Muzzy, W., & Kilpatrick, D. G. (2010). Prevalence and correlates of emotional, physical, sexual, and financial abuse and potential neglect in the United States: The National Elder Mistreatment Study. *American Journal of Public Health, 100*(2), 292–297. doi:10.2105/AJPH.2009.163089

Baker, A. A. (1975). Granny-battering. *Modern Geriatrics, 5,* 20–24.

Brown, A. S. (1989). A survey on elder abuse at one Native American tribe. *Journal of Elder Abuse & Neglect, 1*(2), 17–38. doi:10.1300/J084v01n02_03

Bureau of Indian Affairs. (2014). What we do. Retrieved from http://bia.gov/WhatWeDo/index.htm

Burston, G. R. (1975, September 6). Letter: Granny-battering. *British Medical Journal, 3,* 592. Retrieved from https://www.ncbi.nlm.nih.gov/pmc/articles/PMC1674523/pdf/brmedj01463-0050b.pdf

Butler, R. N. (1975). *Why survive? Being old in America.* New York, NY: Harper & Row.

Butler, R. N. (2008). *The longevity revolution: The benefits and challenges of living a long life.* New York, NY: PublicAffairs.

Choi, N. G., & Mayer, J. (2000). Elder abuse, neglect, and exploitation Risk factors and prevention strategies. *Journal of Gerontological Social Work, 33*(2), 5–25. doi:10.1300/J083v33n02_02

Hickey, T., & Douglass, R. L. (1981). Neglect and abuse of older family members: Professionals' perspectives and case experiences. *Gerontologist, 21*(2), 171–176. doi: 10.1093/geront/21.2.171

Holkup, P. A., Tripp-Reimer, T., Salois, E. M., & Weinert, C. (2004). Community-based participatory research: An approach to intervention research with a Native American community. *Advances in Nursing Science, 27*(3), 162–175. doi:10.1097/00012272-200407000-00002

Ingram, E. M. (2003). Expert panel recommendations on elder mistreatment using a public health framework. *Journal of Elder Abuse & Neglect, 15*(2), 45–65. doi:10.1300/J084v15n02_03

Kate's Bookshelf. (2014, March). Word of the day: Ism (Joycelyn Elders). Retrieved from https://katesbookshelf.wordpress.com/2014/03

Lachs, M. S., & Pillemer, K. (2004). Elder abuse. *Lancet, 364,* 1263–1272. doi:10.1016/ S0140-6736(04)17144-4

Lachs, M. S., Williams, C., O'Brien, S., Hurst, L., & Horwitz, R. (1998). Risk factors for reported elder abuse and neglect: A nine-year observational cohort study. *The Gerontologist, 37*(4), 469–474.

Lachs, M. S., Williams, C. S., O'Brien, S., Pillemer, K. A., & Charlson, M. E. (1998). The mortality of elder mistreatment. *Journal of the American Medical Association, 280*(5), 428–432. doi:10.1001/jama.280.5.428

Laumann, E. O., Leitsch, S. A., & Waite, L. J. (2008). Elder mistreatment in the United States: Prevalence estimates from a nationally representative study. *Journals of Gerontology. Series B: Psychological Sciences and Social Sciences, 63*(4), S248–S254. doi: 10.1093/geronb/63.4.S248

Mann, J. M., Gostin, L., Gruskin, S., Brennan, T., Lazzarini, Z., & Fineberg, H. V. (1994). *Health and human rights* (Vol. 1). Boston, MA: Harvard School of Public Health, Center for Health and Human Rights. Retrieved from https://cdn2.sph .harvard.edu/wp-content/uploads/sites/125/2014/03/4-Mann.pdf

Mercy, J. A., Rosenberg, M. L., Powell, K. E., Broome, C. V., & Roper, W. L. (1993). Public health policy for preventing violence. *Health Affairs, 12*(4), 7–29. doi:10.1377/hlthaff.12.4.7

National Indigenous Elder Justice Initiative. (2014). *Elder abuse codes.* University of North Dakota: Author. Retrieved from http://www.nieji.org/codes

Navarro, A. E., Wilber, K. H., Yonashiro, J., & Homeier, D. C. (2010). Do we really need another meeting? Lessons from the Los Angeles County Elder Abuse Forensic Center. *The Gerontologist, 50*(5), 702–711. doi:10.1093/geront/gnq018.

Perel-Levin, S. (2008). *Discussing screening for elder abuse at primary health care level.* World Health Organization, Ageing and Life Courses. (Based on the MSc dissertation by the same author under the supervision of Philippa Sully: *Interprofessional practice: Society, violence and practice,* St. Bartholomew School of Nursing & Midwifery). Retrieved from http://www.who.int/ageing/publications/ Discussing_Elder_Abuseweb.pdf

Podnieks, E., & Thomas, C. (2016). Consequences of elder abuse and self neglect. In X. Dong (Ed.), *Elder abuse: Research, practice and policy.* New York, NY: Springer International..

Public Health Agency of Canada. (2012). *Elder abuse in Canada: A gender-based analysis.* Division of Aging and Seniors. Retrieved from http://publications.gc .ca/collections/collection_2012/aspc-phac/HP10-21-2012-eng.pdf

Ramsey-Klawsnik, H., & Heisler, C. (2014). Polyvictimization in later life. *Victimization of the Elderly and Disabled, 17*(1), 3–4, 15–16. Retrieved from http://www.napsa-now.org/wp-content/uploads/2016/08/701-Polyvictimization -in-Later-Life.pdf

Roberto, K. A. & Teaster, P. B. (2017). Theorizing elder abuse. In X. Dong (Ed.), *Elder abuse: Research, practice, and policy* (pp. 21–41). New York, NY: Springer Science. doi: 10.1007/978-3-319-47504-2

Schiamberg, L. B., Barboza, G. G., Oehmke, J., Zhang, Z., Griffore, R. J., Weatherill, R. P., . . . & Post, L. A. (2011). Elder abuse in nursing homes: An ecological perspective. *Journal of Elder Abuse & Neglect, 23*(2), 190–211. doi:10.1080/089 46566.2011.558798

Second World Assembly on Ageing. (2002). *Political declaration and Madrid International Plan of action on ageing, Madrid, Spain, 8–12 April 2002.* New York, NY: United Nations. Retrieved from http://www.un.org/en/events/pastevents/pdfs/Madrid_plan.pdf

Teaster, P. B., Otto, J. M., Dugar, T. A., Mendiondo, M. S., Abner, E. L., & Cecil, K. A. (2006). *The 2004 survey of state Adult Protective Services: Abuse of adults 60 years of age and older.* Washington, DC: National Center on Elder Abuse, Administration on Aging.

Teaster, P. B., Roberto, K. A., & Dugar, T. A. (2006). Intimate partner violence of rural aging women. *Family Relations, 55,* 636–648. doi:10.1111/j.1741-3729.2006.00432.x

United Nations General Assembly. (2016). *Protecting humanity from future health crises: Report of the High-Level Panel on the Global Response to Health Crises.* New York, NY: United Nations. Retrieved from http://www.un.org/ga/search/view_doc.asp?symbol=A/70/723

INDEX

Printed in the United States
By Bookmasters